COPD
ASTHMA
and Other Lung Disorders

Diagnosis & Treatments

2018 Report

A Special Report published
by the editors of *HealthNews*
in cooperation with
Duke Health
Duke Division of Pulmonary, Allergy,
and Critical Care Medicine

COPD, Asthma, and Other Lung Disorders: Diagnosis & Treatments

Consulting Editor: Joseph A. Govert, MD, Duke Division of Pulmonary, Allergy, and Critical Care Medicine, Duke Health

Author: Holly Strawbridge
Group Director, Belvoir Media Group: Jay Roland
Content Director, Belvoir Media Group: Larry Canale
Creative Director, Belvoir Media Group: Judi Crouse
Belvoir Editor: Kate Brophy
Production: Mary Francis McGavic

Publisher, Belvoir Media Group: Timothy H. Cole

ISBN: 978-1-879620-90-2

To order additional copies of this report or for customer service questions, please call 877-300-0253, or write to Health Special Reports, 535 Connecticut Avenue, Norwalk, CT 06854-1713.

This publication is intended to provide readers with accurate and timely medical news and information. It is not intended to give personal medical advice, which should be obtained directly from a physician. We regret that we cannot respond to individual inquiries about personal health matters.

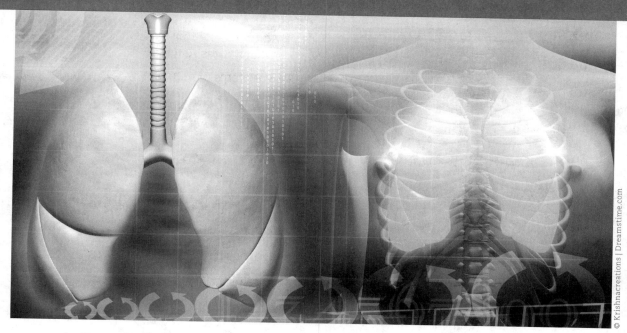

© Krishnacreations | Dreamstime.com

About Duke Medicine

The youngest of the nation's leading medical centers, Duke Medicine has grown since its establishment in 1930 into one of the country's largest clinical and biomedical research institutions. Its health system offers every level of service to more than 1.4 million patients every year, from prevention and primary care to the most sophisticated specialty services. Its nationally top-ranked programs include cancer, cardiology, geriatrics, gynecology, ophthalmology, orthopedics, pulmonology, and urology. The School of Medicine ranks among the nation's top five in grant funding from the National Institutes of Health. In 2003 it forged an education and research collaboration with the National University of Singapore, matriculating the first class of medical students to the Duke-NUS Graduate Medical School Singapore in 2007. Duke is home to the nation's largest and oldest academic clinical research organization—the Duke Clinical Research Institute—which bolsters Duke's comprehensive research programs in areas ranging from cancer and heart disease to the basic sciences and health policy research.

Duke Division of Pulmonary, Allergy, and Critical Care Medicine

Duke's Division of Pulmonary, Allergy, and Critical Care Medicine delivers the most advanced evaluation, diagnosis, and treatment services available to patients suffering from a wide variety of lung diseases and respiratory ailments. An international referral center for patients with pulmonary vascular diseases, Duke also maintains one of the most successful and busiest lung transplantation programs in the country, as well as a highly respected pulmonary rehabilitation program. It is ranked among the nation's top 10 programs by *U.S. News & World Report.*

TABLE OF CONTENTS

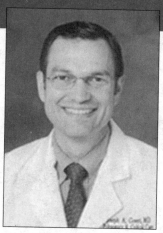

Joseph A. Govert, MD,
Consulting Editor
Duke Division of Pulmonary,
Allergy, and Critical Care
Medicine
Duke Health

Having a lung disorder like chronic obstructive pulmonary disease (COPD), asthma, or pneumonia can be frightening. With every breath we take, we depend on our lungs to deliver life-sustaining oxygen to our bodies—so if you struggle to breathe normally, cough, wheeze, or feel very tired, it's important to find out the cause. It may be something relatively benign, such as a cold. But if it is a more serious disease, like COPD or asthma, getting an early diagnosis and treatment can help you breathe easier and improve your quality of life.

This report covers obstructive lung diseases and lung infections. Obstructive lung diseases include COPD, asthma, and bronchiectasis. Because these obstructive lung diseases produce similar symptoms, making a correct diagnosis can be challenging. Adding to the difficulty is the fact that these conditions can overlap—for example, a person with asthma can acquire chronic bronchitis and/or emphysema, especially if he or she smokes, and this can make it hard to distinguish between asthma and COPD. Bronchiectasis is a less common but often more severe obstructive airway disease that resembles severe bronchitis.

COPD, which encompasses the two conditions emphysema and chronic bronchitis, can't be cured. Smoking is the primary cause of COPD. Fortunately, the rate of smoking is on the decline in the United States, but for those who have symptomatic COPD despite stopping smoking, there are medications that help reduce symptoms and may reduce the risk of flare-ups and hospitalization. Over the last few years, the Food and Drug Administration has approved several new medications and combinations of medications that open narrowed airways in people with COPD. Research is underway to better understand who is at greatest risk for the disease, and to find even more effective future treatments.

Asthma can strike people at just about any age. It is generally not as life threatening as COPD, but getting the right treatment is essential. For people with severe asthma, new types of drugs called biologic agents, which target the cells that cause inflammation in the airways, may revolutionize treatment.

Another set of lung diseases is caused by infections. Germs are on surfaces all around us, and in the air we breathe. The body generally has effective mechanisms for filtering out these germs—but sometimes germs enter the lungs and cause infections like influenza (more commonly called the flu), and pneumonia. The best defense against the flu, and for older adults against pneumonia, is vaccination. Tuberculosis, which used to be more common, is now rare in the U.S., although it remains a major worldwide health problem.

I hope you enjoy reading this report, and find it helpful in increasing your understanding of obstructive lung diseases and lung infections.

Sincerely,

Joseph A. Govert, MD

Joseph A. Govert, MD

HOW THE LUNGS WORK

To understand lung diseases, you need to understand how normal lungs work. The main function of the lungs is to take in oxygen, and get rid of carbon dioxide. Oxygen that flows into your lungs moves into the bloodstream and travels throughout your body, providing every cell with this basic element needed for survival. Carbon dioxide, a gaseous waste product of bodily processes, makes the opposite journey, moving from the cells into the bloodstream and traveling to the lungs. From there it is expelled from the body with every exhalation. Because oxygen and carbon dioxide travel in the bloodstream, the lungs and other organs of the respiratory system must work in concert with the heart, blood, and blood vessels (called the cardiovascular system).

Inside the Lungs

The lungs consist of two large, spongy organs divided into sections called lobes. The right lung has three lobes, and the left lung has two. Inside the lungs is a branching system of progressively smaller tubes (called bronchial tubes), which end in air sacs. Oxygen and carbon dioxide travel through these tubes (see Box 1-1, "How the Lungs Work").

The system of bronchial tubes looks like the branches of a tree. The main trunk is the trachea, and it branches into two large tubes called the right and left mainstem bronchi, each of which leads into one of the two lungs. These bronchi branch off into smaller and smaller tubes called bronchioles. The trachea and the bronchial tubes (bronchi and bronchioles) are often referred to as "airways."

When air (which contains oxygen) is breathed in through the mouth and nose, it passes through the voice box (larynx) and enters the windpipe (trachea), the opening of which is at the back of the throat. Air then travels down the trachea into the bronchial tubes in the lungs.

Oxygen In and Carbon Dioxide Out

At the end of the bronchioles are clusters of tiny air sacs that look like bunches of grapes. These are called alveoli, and there are millions of them. When you inhale, these sacs expand as they fill

BOX 1-1

How the Lungs Work

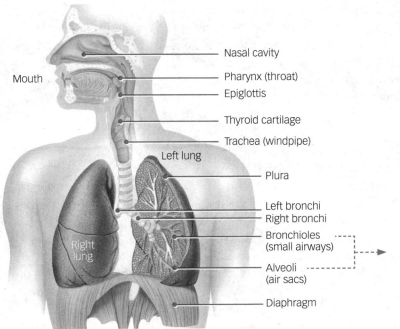

- Mouth
- Nasal cavity
- Pharynx (throat)
- Epiglottis
- Thyroid cartilage
- Trachea (windpipe)
- Left lung
- Plura
- Left bronchi
- Right bronchi
- Bronchioles (small airways)
- Alveoli (air sacs)
- Right lung
- Diaphragm

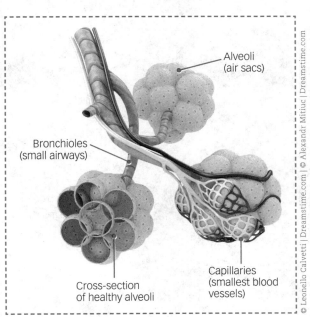

- Alveoli (air sacs)
- Bronchioles (small airways)
- Cross-section of healthy alveoli
- Capillaries (smallest blood vessels)

© Leonello Calvetti | Dreamstime.com | © Alexandr Mitiuc | Dreamstime.com

BOX 1-2

Exchanging Carbon Dioxide for Oxygen in the Lungs

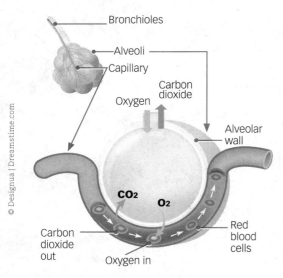

The transfer of oxygen into the bloodstream (from inhaled air) and the transfer out of waste carbon dioxide (from blood) into the lungs occur in the alveoli.

BOX 1-3

The Role of the Diaphragm in Breathing

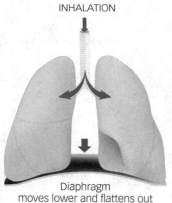

INHALATION

Diaphragm moves lower and flattens out

INHALATION: During inhalation, the diaphragm contracts, meaning it moves lower and flattens out. This causes the chest cavity to enlarge, which reduces pressure and allows air to be drawn into the lungs.

EXHALATION

Diaphragm relaxes and moves back up.

EXHALATION: Exhalation occurs when the diaphragm relaxes and moves back up. Air is pushed out of the lungs by the elasticity of the lungs and chest wall.

with air. When you breathe out, the air sacs deflate. The alveoli have very thin walls, and are surrounded by capillaries (the smallest blood vessels). Where the alveoli and capillaries meet, gas exchange takes place (see Box 1-2, "Exchanging Carbon Dioxide for Oxygen in the Lungs"). Oxygen moves across the walls of the alveoli and enters the tiny capillaries, where it is absorbed into red blood cells. This "oxygenated" blood begins its journey to the heart, and then the rest of the body. At the same time, carbon dioxide from the blood in the capillaries passes into the alveoli. From there, it is expelled from the body through exhalation. This exchange of gases takes just a fraction of a second.

The Process of Breathing

Most people take 12 to 20 breaths every minute. This occurs automatically, but you can also consciously control your breathing, making it faster or slower and even holding your breath for a brief period. The automatic function of breathing is controlled by the brain stem (the lower part of the brain that connects to the spinal cord), along with other functions necessary for survival, including digestion, heart rate, and blood pressure. When the brain senses that there is too little oxygen or too much carbon dioxide, it sends signals to increase the speed and depth of breathing. Because active cells (including muscle cells) require more oxygen for energy and produce more carbon dioxide, breathing increases with exercise and slows down during rest.

The mechanical process of breathing depends on several muscles, the largest of which is the diaphragm. This dome-shaped muscle is positioned just below the lungs, and separates the chest cavity from the abdomen (see Box 1-3, "The Role of the Diaphragm in Breathing"). During inhalation, the diaphragm flattens out, causing the chest cavity to enlarge. This reduces pressure in the chest cavity and allows air to be drawn into the lungs. When the diaphragm relaxes, air is pushed out of the lungs. Other muscles also are at work during the process of breathing. When these muscles are working most efficiently, more air is pulled into lower lobes of the lung.

The Role of the Heart and Circulatory System

There are two types of blood vessels: Veins carry blood toward the heart, and arteries carry it away from the heart. Arteries bring blood that contains oxygen (oxygenated) to the tissues of the body, and veins carry blood that is void of oxygen (deoxygenated) and full of carbon dioxide back to the heart. Through the heart's pumping action, blood that has been depleted of oxygen and contains carbon dioxide is sent from the heart into the lungs. Once gas exchange takes place in the lungs, the newly oxygenated blood returns to the heart. From there, the heart pumps the oxygenated blood into the aorta (the main artery) and out into the branching system of smaller and smaller arteries to reach the rest of the body (see Box 1-4, "Blood Flow: Heart and Lungs").

Protective Mechanisms of Bronchial Tubes

Bronchi and bronchioles are essentially tubes with muscular walls. Lining the inside of these tubes are several layers of tissue. The innermost lining is called the mucosa, and it contains cells that help protect the lungs. One type of cell in the mucosa produces the sticky substance known as mucus. The mucosa also contains cells with hair-like projections called cilia. Mucus serves many useful functions. For example, it traps bacteria, pollen, and other particles that have been inhaled. These are then swept away from the lungs and up toward the mouth by the motion of the tiny cilia and cleared away, mostly through swallowing. Coughing can also get rid of mucus. When you get a cold or flu, excess mucus is created. The mucus (also called sputum) that comes up when you cough is helping to eliminate the infectious agent. Once the infection is gone, mucus production returns to its normal state and coughing eventually stops.

The bronchial tubes are surrounded by bands of muscle. Certain cells in the lining of the bronchial tubes have receptors that stimulate these muscles to contract and relax. For example, a type of receptor called a beta-adrenergic receptor causes muscles to relax, which widens the airway, making it easier to breathe. Another type of receptor, called a cholinergic receptor, causes the muscles to contract, narrowing the airway and making it harder to breathe. Normally, this keeps irritants out of the lungs. For people with obstructive lung diseases, this narrowing can make it even more difficult to breathe.

BOX 1-4

Blood Flow: Heart and Lungs

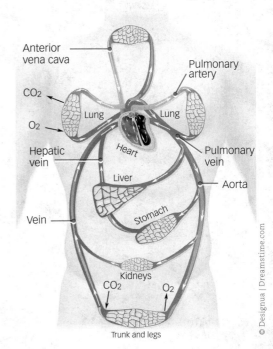

© Designua | Dreamstime.com

The heart has four chambers: two ventricles and two atria (the plural of atrium).

Deoxygenated blood returning to the heart through the veins enters the right atrium.

From there it moves through a valve called the tricuspid valve into the right ventricle (the function of heart valves is to keep blood flowing in the right direction between chambers).

The blood then enters the pulmonary artery, which brings it into the lungs.

Blood from the lungs, which has received oxygen, returns to the heart by entering the left atrium.

From there, the blood flows through the mitral valve into the left ventricle.

The oxygenated blood then flows through the aortic valve into the main artery of the body (the aorta), and from there the blood is carried throughout the body.

OBSTRUCTIVE LUNG DISEASES

Just as the name implies, obstructive lung diseases stem from some abnormality that interferes with normal airflow into and out of the lungs. They include COPD, asthma, and bronchiectasis. The Centers for Disease Control and Prevention (CDC) report that about 15.7 million Americans have been diagnosed with COPD, and millions more may be undiagnosed (see Box 2-1, "Women More Likely to Suffer Severe COPD"). Additionally, 25.7 percent, including children, have asthma. Bronchiectasis is far less common but can be very disabling.

Obstructive lung diseases can cause

- Chronic cough
- Difficulty breathing
- Periodic wheezing

While the symptoms of obstructive lung diseases can be similar, the causes and treatment often differ.

CHRONIC OBSTRUCTIVE PULMONARY DISEASE (COPD)

Chronic obstructive pulmonary disease (COPD) used to describe two conditions—emphysema and chronic bronchitis—that make it difficult to breathe in and out. Today, COPD is simply described as a disease characterized by chronic airflow limitation caused by small airway disease and/or destruction of the lung tissues involved in exchanging oxygen for carbon dioxide (see Box 2-2, "Out With the Old Terms, In With the New"). These problems may be present in different degrees and evolve at different rates. Nevertheless, the changes cause breathlessness (dyspnea), chronic cough, and sputum production. COPD is most often caused by significant exposure to noxious particles and gases, primarily tobacco smoke. The course of COPD may be punctuated by periods of worsening symptoms called exacerbations.

COPD can be prevented, but it cannot be cured. Fortunately, treatment to make breathing easier and prolong life is available for those with the disease.

What Takes Place in COPD?

Inhaling noxious gases or particles causes inflammation in the lungs. When inflammation becomes chronic, changes in lung tissue occur. The airways become narrowed. The bronchi, bronchioles, and alveoli are normally very elastic, which means they stretch and recoil during the process of breathing. In COPD this elasticity is reduced. As a result, the airways and alveoli are no longer able to bounce back to their original shape, especially during exhalation. Some of the airways collapse, preventing some alveoli from deflating and causing air to get trapped in the lungs. This causes parts of the lung to become enlarged, or hyperinflated. Destruction of the alveoli also hampers the exchange of oxygen and carbon dioxide. This leads to too little oxygen and too much carbon dioxide in the blood.

The presence of harmful substances also sparks the increased production of mucus in the bronchial tubes. Under normal circumstances, once the intruder has been eliminated, inflammation and excess mucus production subside. But in people with COPD, the inflammation and excess mucus production persist. In addition, inhaled tobacco smoke damages the hair-like cilia that normally help to sweep mucus out of the lungs and expel toxic substances. Constant inflammation in the airways, an overabundance of mucus, and decreased ability to clear the mucus cause the passageways in the bronchi to narrow. This can cause difficulty breathing and, typically, a chronic cough.

What Causes COPD?

The primary cause of COPD is smoking, but long-term exposure to air pollution, dust, or certain chemicals also may cause or contribute to it.

A diet that is rich in fiber (from whole grains, whole fruits, vegetables, beans, brown rice, and nuts), and low in red meat, refined

COPD is currently the fourth-leading cause of death in the world, but is projected to be the third-leading cause by 2020.

NEW FINDING BOX 2-2

Out With the Old Terms, In With the New

The Global Initiative on Obstructive Lung Disease (GOLD) is an organization that works with healthcare professionals and public health officials to raise awareness of COPD and improve prevention and treatment for patients worldwide.

In 2017, GOLD updated its consensus report on the diagnosis, prevention, and management of COPD to reflect new literature and new thinking about the disease. This report includes many changes, starting with elimination of the terms "chronic bronchitis" and "emphysema." GOLD's reasoning is that the characteristics of these two diseases vary from person to person and evolve at different rates over time. Moreover, the destruction of tissue from emphysema is only one of several abnormalities present in COPD, and only a minority of patients with COPD have the inflammation associated with chronic bronchitis.

Today, GOLD explains what COPD is by saying that the chronic airflow limitation characteristic of COPD is caused by a mixture of small airways disease (obstructive bronchiolitis) and the destruction of lung tissue (emphysema).

Global Initiative for Chronic Obstructive Lung Disease, 2017 grains, and sugar may help keep the lungs healthy and reduce the chances of getting COPD for both smokers and nonsmokers. However, it is unknown whether changing fiber intake improves lung function in patients who already have COPD.

Smoking

COPD most often affects people age 40 and older who have smoked a pack of cigarettes per day for 10 or more years. Pipe and cigar smoking also can decrease lung function and increase the chance of COPD, even in people who have never smoked cigarettes. So can smoking water pipes or marijuana.

Smokers who have a family history of COPD are at particularly high risk. For some people, exposure to secondhand smoke can cause respiratory symptoms and possibly COPD. Exposure to secondhand smoke in childhood appears to increase the risk for developing COPD in adulthood. In a 2016 study, middle-aged people whose mothers were heavy smokers (more than 20 cigarettes a day) were more than twice as likely to have lung impairment indicative of COPD than people whose mothers had not smoked.

People who have quit smoking are still at increased risk of eventually being diagnosed with COPD. But stopping smoking significantly reduces the chances of getting COPD, as well as other lung and heart diseases. Smokers with COPD who stop smoking slow the progression of their COPD. Smoking also increases the risk for lung cancer, but this risk declines when a person stops smoking, and continues to decline the longer they go without smoking.

E-cigarettes were introduced into the United States in 2006 as a supposedly safe alternative to tobacco cigarettes. However, it remains uncertain whether they actually are safe. Despite the lack of long-term research, some studies suggest these products may not be as benign as they seem. E-cigarettes typically contain nicotine, a flavoring, and a solvent. According to one study, they also contain additives with unknown health risks (see Box 2-3, "Want a Puff of Insecticide?").

More studies are underway to assess whether e-cigarettes and other electronic nicotine delivery systems (ENDS) help with smoking cessation. To date, the results of randomized, controlled clinical trials is mixed. As far as safety goes, studies have linked the use of ENDS to changes in airflow that precede COPD, daytime cough, phlegm production, headache, dry mouth, vertigo, and nausea.

In 2016, the Food and Drug Administration began regulating the manufacture, packaging, labeling, advertising, sale, and distribution of ENDS. All ENDS products must carry a warning that the product contains nicotine, and that nicotine is addictive. They are not required to say what other chemicals they contain.

Genetics

Since not all smokers develop COPD, experts believe that a combination of smoking and genetic factors may be at work in those who do get the disease. With the exception of the alpha-1 antitrypsin gene, the specific genes that may be involved are not known, but researchers have begun to identify possible candidates.

Occupational Exposures

Long-term exposure to various kinds of chemicals, fumes, and dust can also harm the lungs and cause COPD.

Several occupations potentially expose workers to inhalants that, when breathed in over long periods of time, can damage the lungs. For example, agricultural workers may be exposed to gases and organic dusts generated by cotton, flax, hay, and grains, or fertilizers and pesticides. Cotton textile workers may inhale cotton dust. Flourmill workers and bakers may breathe in flour and other grain particles. Exposure to coal mine dust over a full working lifetime, even at the federally mandated limits imposed in 1972, produces a cumulative exposure that appears to increase the risk for COPD.

Occupational exposure to chemicals, fumes, and dust can also lead to asthma. It is often very difficult to distinguish occupational asthma from occupation-induced COPD. The primary treatment for either condition, however, is removal of the offending exposure. Similar medications are used to treat both conditions.

Air Pollution

Whether outdoor air pollution from sources such as automobile, factory, and power plant emissions can cause COPD is uncertain. But there is some evidence that it damages the lungs. One study found that people who lived near major roadways (less than 109 yards away) and were exposed over a long period of time to the tiny particles in automobile exhaust had poorer lung function and a faster decline in lung function over time than people living more than one-quarter mile away from a major road.

Another type of outdoor air pollution is ozone. In the upper atmosphere, ozone protects against harmful ultraviolet radiation. When present at ground level, ozone (which forms when exhaust from tailpipes, coal-fired power plants, and other sources mixes with oxygen) is a pollutant. One study found that increased levels of ground-level ozone correlated with increased risk of dying from respiratory illnesses, including COPD. For people who already have COPD, exposure to high levels of outdoor air pollution can exacerbate their condition.

Indoor air pollution from heating and cooking stoves used in poorly ventilated dwellings is a primary cause of COPD for women who live in developing countries. In the U.S. and other developed countries, studies have found that exposure to wood smoke may increase risk for smokers. One study found that smokers who are consistently exposed to both wood smoke (from a fireplace, wood-burning stove, or in the air) and tobacco smoke are at greater risk for COPD than people exposed to just one of these types of smoke. In addition, people who already have COPD and are exposed to both types of smoke experience more frequent and severe symptoms.

Alpha-1 Antitrypsin Deficiency

In a small number of people, COPD is caused by a hereditary disorder called alpha-1 antitrypsin deficiency. Alpha-1 antitrypsin is a protein that prevents an enzyme called neutrophil elastase from damaging the alveoli. People with alpha-1 antitrypsin deficiency lack this protein, and about 75 percent of adults with this deficiency develop COPD. This genetic disorder is most commonly seen in individuals of Northern European ancestry. People with this deficiency who smoke are at particularly high risk of developing severe lung disease, often at a relatively young age.

Symptoms of COPD

COPD often develops gradually over time, making it difficult to diagnose until it is quite advanced. The lungs, with over 300 million alveoli, have an amazing capacity. Not all of these alveoli are used for the day-to-day work of normal breathing. As we age, we lose some of this excess capacity, but in the absence of a lung disease, the lungs continue to function very well.

Because most people never use their full lung capacity, diminished lung function often is not noticed in the early stages of COPD. As the disease gets worse, people may become less active without realizing their lung function is compromised. They may be unaware of the extent of their limitations, and also unaware that these limitations are due to a lung disease. At some point—often at relatively low levels of exertion—the body is no longer able to compensate, and symptoms become impossible to ignore.

The salient symptoms of COPD include:
- Progressive shortness of breath, particularly with exertion (walking, climbing stairs)
- A cough that doesn't go away
- Sputum (mucus) production, especially in the morning
- Wheezing (a whistling or squeaky sound when you breathe)
- Chest tightness
- In severe disease, fatigue, weight loss, anorexia, fainting during coughing spelling, ankle swelling, depression, anxiety

Shortness of breath is the symptom that drives most people with undiagnosed COPD to see a doctor. At first, shortness of breath is only noticeable with exertion, but eventually breathlessness hampers routine daily activities such as washing, dressing, and cooking. Chronic cough may at first be intermittent, but later may occur every day. For people with COPD, it is common to cough up small quantities of sputum. As the disease gets worse, the sputum may become thicker. Wheezing and chest tightness may or may not be present every day, but often become prominent when people with COPD catch a cold.

The frequency and severity of episodes of coughing and shortness of breath increase as the disease worsens. Fatigue and weakness are common complaints. Weight loss may occur in the more advanced stages of the disease, along with morning headaches due to a build-up of carbon dioxide in the blood overnight.

Having a chronic cough and coughing up sputum when there is no identifiable reason, such as a cold or flu, is not normal. It is important to see a doctor during the early signs of lung disease, because effective treatments are available to assist with breathing and improve quality of life. In addition, smokers who learn they have developed lung disease early in the course of the disease may be able to stop smoking

---

NEW FINDING   BOX 2-4

COPD Flare-Ups May Worsen Lung Function

A recent study reports that sudden flare-ups of symptoms (exacerbations) may accelerate loss of lung function in people with COPD, and especially those in the mild stages.

Researchers examined data from about 2,000 current or former smokers, who had had their lung function tested at the start of the study and five years later. The researchers also collected data on exacerbations. They found that 35 percent of participants reported at least one exacerbation. Among study participants with diagnosed COPD, having exacerbations resulted in excess loss of lung function. The greatest excess loss of lung function associated with exacerbations was seen in people with mild COPD.

American Journal of Respiratory and Critical Care Medicine, February 1, 2017

before the disease becomes more serious. Many people with COPD wait until breathing has become a chore and their quality of life is seriously compromised before they consult a doctor. While smoking cessation is still important at that point, it is less effective in preventing serious complications of COPD.

Studies have shown that many current and former smokers display symptoms of COPD even though their lung function tests do not meet the criteria to be diagnosed with the disease. It is still unclear whether their lung function will eventually worsen to the point where they are diagnosed, or whether they should receive treatment.

Exacerbations

Exacerbations are sudden flare-ups of COPD symptoms beyond normal day-to-day variations. Common features include increased breathlessness along with wheezing, chest tightness, increased cough and sputum, change of the color of sputum, and fever. Serious exacerbations may require hospitalization. Studies have found that exacerbations of COPD may speed up loss of lung function, especially for people with mild COPD (see Box 2-4, "COPD Flare-Ups May Worsen Lung Function," on page 14).

Where you live may make a difference in how often you have an exacerbation. One study found that people with COPD who live in communities that ban smoking in public places were 22 percent less likely to be hospitalized for COPD exacerbations than those living in communities that do not have such laws.

In 30 percent of exacerbations, no cause is identified but a recent retrospective study suggests that blood clots in the lungs (pulmonary emboli, or PE) may be responsible in some cases (see Box 2-5, "The Role of PE in COPD Exacerbations").

Distinguishing COPD From Asthma

The symptoms of COPD and asthma can be similar, especially in the early stages of COPD, and the two conditions can coexist. Therefore, for some people, especially those who smoke, it may be difficult to make an accurate diagnosis. However, there are some distinguishing characteristics. For example, asthma can affect people at any age, while COPD rarely occurs before age 40. Other key differences between COPD and asthma are listed in Box 2-6, "Differences Between COPD and Asthma."

One major difference between asthma and COPD relates to the reversibility of the condition. In COPD, the damage to the airways is not fully reversible. Rather, it is permanent, and gets progressively worse. The airway narrowing in asthma, on the other hand, is usually reversible. In addition, an asthma attack is generally sparked by a trigger, such as an allergic reaction, exposure to the cold, or exercise. Doctors can simulate an asthma trigger with an inhaled drug called methacholine. This drug causes the airways to spasm, which will be detected on a test of breathing function (spirometry, see Chapter 3). A positive result of this test indicates asthma is probably the cause of the person's symptoms. However, this is not 100 percent accurate

NEW FINDING   BOX 2-5

The Role of PE in COPD Exacerbations

Acute exacerbations of COPD are caused by increased inflammation in the lungs, but the reason for these sudden increases remains unknown in about 30 percent of cases.

Knowing that inflammation can also trigger the formation of blood clots, researchers searched for studies that included patients with acute exacerbations of COPD and pulmonary embolisms (PE, or blood clots in the lungs). PE were found in 16.1 percent of 880 patients. The researchers suggested that physicians be on the lookout for PE in patients with acute exacerbations of COPD, particularly when no infection is present. Such PE may require treatment with anticoagulants.

Chest, March 2017

BOX 2-6

Differences Between COPD and Asthma

COPD
• Usually begins after age 40
• Symptoms get worse with advancing age
• Occurs in people with a history of smoking
• Limitation in airflow is not reversible

Asthma
• Usually begins in childhood
• Symptoms can vary from day to day
• Symptoms often occur at night or in the early morning
• Allergy, rhinitis, and/or eczema are usually present
• Family history of asthma
• Limitation in airflow is largely reversible with medication

Global Initiative for Chronic Obstructive Lung Disease

PAD More Prevalent in People With COPD

In a study of 2,088 patients with all stages of COPD, 8.8 percent were found to have peripheral arterial disease (PAD) caused by atherosclerosis (narrowing) in the leg arteries. This compared with only 5.9 percent of patients without COPD. The patients with COPD and PAD were far less able to finish the six-minute walk test, reported worse health status, and were not able to function as well as people without COPD and PAD.

American Journal of Respiratory and Critical Care Medicine, January 15, 2017

because a person with chronic bronchitis also may have a positive result on this test.

People with asthma (especially those who smoke) can develop a chronic cough, and can develop COPD. It may not always be possible to make a clear distinction between asthma and COPD. People suspected of having both COPD and asthma will likely need to see a specialist to confirm the diagnosis. Treatment can be challenging because the two conditions are generally treated differently. Each patient is different—therefore, treatment should be individualized.

COPD and Other Health Conditions

COPD may be a lung disease, but most people with COPD also have other significant chronic diseases. These commonly include skeletal muscle disease, cardiovascular disease, metabolic syndrome, osteoporosis, depress, anxiety and lung cancer. According to the Global Initiative for Chronic Obstructive Lung Disease, the existence of COPD may actually increase the risk for other diseases, lung cancer in particular.

Very severe COPD may cause a type of high blood pressure in the lungs called pulmonary hypertension. Because the lungs are not working efficiently, the heart must work harder to pump blood into the lungs. This can cause high blood pressure in the arteries that bring blood into the lungs. Severe COPD also appears to increase the risk for heart attack, stroke, and heart failure. Heart function may be diminished in patients with COPD, even if they have only mild symptoms. Recently, COPD was found to be associated with peripheral arterial disease (PAD), a form of cardiovascular disease in the legs (see Box 2-7, "PAD More Prevalent in People with COPD").

Older adults with COPD appear to have an increased risk for a type of mental decline called mild cognitive impairment. They are also more likely to be diagnosed with depression than healthy individuals or those with a different chronic illness (diabetes, for example).

People with COPD are at increased risk for developing shingles, most likely because having COPD weakens the immune system. Shingles is a reactivation of the chicken pox virus that produces a painful rash and can result in lasting nerve damage.

People with COPD are also more likely to catch a cold or the flu, and are more susceptible to getting pneumonia.

DIAGNOSING COPD

COPD and asthma share many of the same symptoms (primarily coughing, wheezing, and shortness of breath), which occur because normal airflow into and out of the lungs is obstructed. This can make it difficult to distinguish between the two conditions, especially in middle- and older-aged adults with a history of smoking. Regardless of the age that these symptoms first appear, it's important to make an accurate diagnosis, because treatment often differs for the two conditions.

The first step is to perform a physical examination, take a detailed medical history, ask about smoking (in adults) and other lifestyle issues, and perform diagnostic tests.

COPD is suspected in anyone with a history of smoking or exposure to environmental irritants who has any of the characteristic symptoms of COPD.

In a patient with symptoms of COPD, or a history of exposure to risk factors for COPD (such as cigarette smoke), spirometry is used to make the diagnosis. It is also used to assess the severity of COPD.

Using the spirometry reading, a patient's COPD is classified by stage: mild, moderate, severe, and very severe (see Box 3-1, "Stages of COPD"). These classifications are based on increasing severity of airflow restriction and symptoms.

In someone with COPD, the amount of air that can be blown out in one second (FEV 1) drops. As the disease worsens, the total amount of air that can be exhaled after inhalation (FVC) also drops.

Tests Used to Diagnose COPD
Spirometry

Spirometry is a lung function test that measures the amount of air you inhale and exhale. In spirometry, the patient takes a deep breath in and then exhales as hard and as long as possible into a hose connected to a machine called a spirometer. The machine measures how fast air is blown out of the lungs, as well as the total amount of air inhaled and exhaled (see Box 3-2, "What a Spirometer Measures," on page 18). The results will be abnormal in someone with COPD.

Generally, after taking a spirometry test, the patient is given a bronchodilator medication to inhale. Then the test is repeated. If results improve after taking a bronchodilator, the patient likely has asthma rather than COPD, since asthma is often reversible. If COPD is present, airflow will continue to be limited, even after taking the drug.

Chest X-Ray

Some patients will be given a chest X-ray to see if the changes consistent with emphysema are present. A chest X-ray can also reveal whether the symptoms might be caused by a condition such as heart failure.

BOX 3-1

Stages of COPD

Stage I: Mild COPD
Spirometry (breathing test) shows mild limitation in airflow (FEV1 greater than 80 percent of predicted). Chronic cough and sputum production may be present. At this stage, the person is often unaware of their impaired lung function.

Stage II: Moderate COPD
Spirometry shows limitation in airflow that is worse than in mild COPD (FEV1 less than 80 percent but greater than 50 percent of predicted). Shortness of breath typically occurs with exertion. Cough and sputum production are more likely than in mild COPD. At this stage, the person may first become aware of a problem with breathing and seek medical advice.

Stage III: Severe COPD
Airflow limitation becomes progressively worse (FEV1 less than 50 percent but greater than 30 percent of predicted). Shortness of breath will increase, even with just a small amount of exertion, and the person will likely feel fatigued. Quality of life often diminishes.

Stage IV: Very severe COPD
Airflow is severely compromised (FEV1 less than 30 percent of predicted, or less than 50 percent of predicted, plus the person has chronic respiratory failure). This may lead to heart problems, such as heart failure. Quality of life is markedly impaired. Exacerbations of the disease may be life threatening.

BOX 3-2

What a Spirometer Measures

The spirometer can be used to take several types of measurements. Some common ones used in the diagnosis and management of obstructive lung diseases are as follows:

- **Forced vital capacity (FVC):** The total amount of air that can forcibly be blown out after inhalation.

- **Forced expiratory volume in 1 second (FEV1):** The amount of air that can be blown out in one second.

- **The ratio of FEV1 to FVC (FEV1/FVC):** In healthy adults, this should be 75 to 80 percent.

- **Peak expiratory flow (PEF):** The speed of air moving out of the lungs at the beginning of an exhalation.

Computed Tomography

Computed tomography (CT) is another noninvasive imaging test that may be used to detect emphysema or bronchiectasis. It also may be used to decide whether a patient with COPD is a candidate for lung surgery.

Arterial Blood Gas Test

An arterial blood gas test may be performed to measure the amount of oxygen and carbon dioxide in the blood. It is used to determine whether there is too little oxygen in the blood (a condition called hypoxemia), or to detect the presence of too much carbon dioxide (called hypercapnia).

Blood Tests

In people younger than age 40 with the characteristic signs and symptoms of COPD, the physician will likely order a blood test to determine if the cause is a genetic condition known as alpha-1 antitrypsin deficiency (see Chapter 2). The test also may be ordered for someone with COPD symptoms who has a strong family history of COPD, or a family history of the enzyme deficiency.

TREATING COPD

Even though COPD cannot be cured, it can be treated. Treatment is aimed at reducing symptoms, preventing the disease from getting worse, improving the ability to exercise, preventing and treating complications, and preventing and treating exacerbations.

For those with COPD who are current smokers, the most important first step is to quit. Smoking cessation helps to slow down the disease, especially in its early stages. People with COPD should also reduce their exposure to secondhand smoke, occupational sources of lung irritants (like dust and chemicals), and indoor and outdoor air pollutants. When outdoor air quality is poor, persons with significant COPD should stay indoors to help reduce symptoms (see Box 4-1, "Minimizing the Effects of Outdoor Air Pollution").

In people with COPD, the parts of the lungs damaged due to emphysema cannot be restored. Therefore, treatment is used to improve function in the parts of the lungs that are still working, and reduce inflammation in the lungs.

In addition to medications, regular physical activity is important for maintaining lung function. For patients with more severe disease, a specialized exercise program called pulmonary rehabilitation has been shown to improve the ability to exercise and engage in basic daily activities with less shortness of breath. In severe disease, oxygen therapy is often required. Some people with advanced COPD may be candidates for lung volume reduction surgery, which may relieve symptoms and can improve quality of life, or lung transplantation. Everyone with COPD should receive immunizations for influenza and pneumonia.

BOX 4-1

Minimizing the Effects of Outdoor Air Pollution

Air pollution can worsen COPD symptoms and trigger asthma attacks.

Air pollution consists of solid particles in the air (called particulate matter), and ozone. Particulate matter is a combination of very small solids, such as dust, ash or soot, and liquid droplets. These particles, which are emitted by wood stoves, diesel-powered trucks and buses, and coal-fired power plants, among other sources, can enter the airways and damage the lungs.

The ozone layer high in the atmosphere acts as a protective filter against the damaging ultraviolet rays of the sun. However, high concentrations of ozone closer to the ground can be a lung irritant. Sunlight combined with hydrocarbons and nitrogen gas (produced by the burning of fuel such as gasoline, diesel, kerosene, oil, or natural gas) produces ground-level ozone.

The Environmental Protection Agency (EPA) created the Air Quality Index (AQI) to inform the public about local air quality and whether air pollution levels pose a possible health concern. Asthma attacks are most likely to occur the day after outdoor pollution levels are high.

The EPA recommends the following steps to reduce exposure to outdoor air pollution when the AQI reports unhealthy levels:

- Stay indoors if possible.
- Go outside only in the early morning or evening (ozone levels tend to be highest in the middle of the day).
- Refrain from strenuous outdoor physical activity while air pollution levels are high, reduce the intensity of the activity, or consider indoor sports.

To learn more about how the AQI works, visit www.epa.gov/airnow.

"State of the Air"

The American Lung Association provides information about air quality on the website State of the Air (www.stateoftheair.org). A "State of the Air" app is available for smartphones and tablets to check ozone and particulate pollution.

BOX 4-2

Bronchodilator Drugs

	Short-Acting (Immediate relief)	Long-Acting (Longer-term relief)
BETA-AGONISTS	• **Albuterol** (ProAir HFA, ProAir RespiClick, Proventil HFA, Ventolin HFA) • **Levalbuterol** (Xopenex) • **Metaproterenol** (Alupent, Metaprel) • **Pirbuterol** (Maxair Autohaler) • **Terbutaline [for asthma only]** (Brethine, Bricamyl, Brethaire, Terbulin)	• **Arformoterol** (Brovana) • **Formoterol** (Foradil, Perforomist [for COPD only]) • **Indacaterol** (Arcapta Neohaler [for COPD only]) • **Olodaterol** (Striverdi Respimat [for COPD only]) • **Salmeterol** (Serevent)
ANTICHOLINERGICS	• **Ipratropium** (Atrovent)	• **Aclidinium [for COPD only]** (Tudorza Pressair) • **Tiotropium** (Spiriva) • **Umeclidinium** (Incruse Ellipta [for COPD only])

Drugs to Treat Obstructive Airway Diseases

Drug therapy is part of the treatment for just about everyone with COPD or asthma. Drug regimens generally include two types of medicines:

- Bronchodilators to open narrowed airways
- Anti-inflammatory drugs (corticosteroids) to reduce inflammation in the lungs.

Various combinations of these medications often are used.

Bronchodilators

Bronchodilators expand the airways, making it easier to breathe and go about daily life. There are two main types of bronchodilators (see Box 4-2, "Bronchodilator Drugs"): beta-agonists and anticholinergics. Each is available in a short-acting and a long-acting formulation. A third type of bronchodilator, theophylline, is an older drug that is used less frequently.

Beta-agonists and anticholinergics can be taken orally, intravenously, or through inhalation. The preferred method for delivering the drugs to people with obstructive airway disease is inhalation. Using an inhaler device, the drug is breathed in and quickly goes to the airway, where it is needed. There are generally fewer side effects with inhaled medications than there are with pills.

To ensure that the correct amount of drug is delivered, proper inhaler technique is needed. Poor technique can result in too little drug reaching the lungs, as well as more side effects due to the drug being deposited in the mouth or the back of the throat.

Beta-Agonists

Beta-agonists activate a receptor on muscles surrounding the bronchial tubes, causing them to relax and allowing the airway to dilate. Short-acting beta-agonists start to work within minutes and last about four to six hours. Long-acting beta-agonists (LABAs) take longer to begin working (about 20 minutes), but last up to 24 hours.

The possible side effects of beta-agonists include headaches, nervousness, dizziness, and shakiness. If side effects occur, they often last only a short time and diminish or resolve completely once the medication is used regularly. If they persist, a different medication, or a lower dose may be prescribed.

Anticholinergics

Anticholinergics block a receptor in the lung to prevent the airways from constricting. This allows the airways to remain open. The short-acting anticholinergic drug ipratropium (Atrovent) starts to work within 15 minutes, and lasts for six to eight hours. Long-acting anticholinergic drugs take 10-20 minutes to start working, and last 12-24 hours.

Possible side effects of ipratropium are coughing, headaches, nausea, heartburn, diarrhea, urinary retention, and constipation, among others. However, they are generally not serious and diminish or go away completely if the medication is stopped. If any side effect is severe, or does not go away, a different medication may be needed.

Anti-Inflammatory Drugs

Anti-inflammatory medications reduce inflammation. Corticosteroids are the most commonly used anti-inflammatory drugs given to people with COPD or asthma to reduce swelling in the bronchial tubes. They can be taken in tablet, liquid, injected, or inhaled form.

Corticosteroids do not work as quickly as bronchodilators: It can take up to a week to notice the effect. The pill form acts faster than the inhaled version, but often causes more side effects.

Corticosteroids

Oral corticosteroids—most commonly prednisone (Deltasone) and predisolone (Medrol)—are generally reserved for treating acute exacerbations of COPD or asthma. Breathing becomes easier, coughing and wheezing subside, and mucus production lessens.

Even though oral corticosteroids have pronounced effects, they are generally only used for a short period of time (a few days to a few weeks). This is because in addition to reducing inflammation, corticosteroids have other effects on the body that can cause unwanted and potentially severe consequences. Taken by mouth in moderate-to-high doses for months or years, corticosteroids can cause bruising of the skin, cataracts, bone thinning (osteoporosis), muscle weakness, hair loss, growth of facial hair in women, mood changes, and weight gain. Anyone who uses oral steroids for long periods of time may also be susceptible to developing high blood pressure and/or diabetes. Moreover, when oral steroids are used for more than a few weeks, the body becomes accustomed to the drug and it cannot be stopped abruptly without adverse effects. Therefore, anyone who takes an oral steroid for several weeks or more must taper off the drug rather than stopping it abruptly.

Inhaled Corticosteroids

Most people with obstructive airway disease who take corticosteroids will use the inhaled form (see Box 4-3, "Inhaled Corticosteroids"). By using an inhaler device, the medication is delivered directly to the lungs. Very little medication travels through the bloodstream, which minimizes side effects. In commonly used doses, inhaled steroids are safe to use over the long term. Possible side effects are a sore throat, hoarse voice, and a yeast infection in the mouth (oral candidiasis). Candidiasis can be avoided by rinsing your mouth with water after each use of the inhaler, or by using a spacer.

As with bronchodilators, proper technique using the inhaler device is critical to the successful delivery of the correct dose of the drug.

Types of Inhalers

Inhalers deliver bronchodilators or corticosteroid medications as a spray, mist, or fine powder. Three types of devices are available to deliver inhaled medications: a metered dose inhaler (MDI), a dry powder inhaler (DPI), and a nebulizer.

Metered Dose Inhalers

An MDI is a small, pressurized canister with a mouthpiece and a metering valve that contains medication. The patient places his or her

BOX 4-3

Inhaled Corticosteroids

- Triamcinolone (Azmacort)
- Beclomethasone (Vanceril, Qvar, Beclovent)
- Flunisolide (AeroBid, AeroBid-M)
- Fluticasone (Flovent)
- Budesonide (Pulmicort)

BOX 4-4

MDI Technique

When using a metered dose inhaler (MDI), proper technique is essential for delivering the correct amount of the prescribed drug. The design of different inhaler devices may vary, so it is important to read the directions carefully before using an inhaler for the first time. Clean your inhaler once a week by following the cleaning directions that came with your device. Also, find out how many puffs of medicine the inhaler contains and keep track of how many you use, so you know when to refill your prescription.

In general, to use an MDI:

1. Remove the cap from the inhaler.
2. Shake the inhaler.

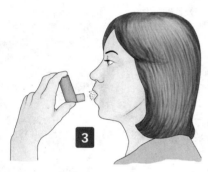

3. Exhale completely.

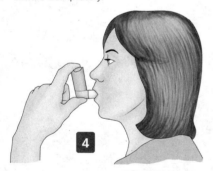

4. Place the mouthpiece of the inhaler (or spacer) in your mouth, with your lips sealed around it.
5. Inhale slowly and deeply while pressing down on the top of the canister to release the medication.
6. Hold your breath for 10 seconds.
7. Exhale.
8. If you need to take another puff of medicine, wait one minute.
9. If the medication is an inhaled steroid, rinse out your mouth. Spit the water out; do not swallow it.
10. Replace the cap on the inhaler.

mouth over the mouthpiece, and then inhales while pushing down on the top of the canister to deliver a precise dose of the medication.

The proper technique for using an MDI inhaler is described in Box 4-4, "MDI Technique." Several common mistakes can lead to too little or too much medication being delivered. For example, some people exhale before the end of the spray, or inhale after the medication is sprayed. Other mistakes include inhaling through the nose instead of the mouth, squeezing the canister twice but only inhaling once, or forgetting to take the cap off the mouthpiece.

Many people find it helpful to use a spacer device with their MDI to improve drug delivery. A spacer is a short tube that is placed between the mouthpiece of the inhaler and your mouth. The medicine enters the tube, and from there it can be inhaled more slowly and deeply. This results in more effective delivery of the medicine to the lungs.

The medication in the MDI canister is suspended in a mixture of substances. One of these is a propellant, which squirts the mixture out of the device and gives it enough momentum to get down into the lungs. The mix also contains preservatives, flavoring agents, and chemicals that help to disperse the drug throughout the lung.

Each inhaler has different directions for washing, drying the mouthpiece, and priming. It's important to follow the instructions that come with the inhaler your doctor has prescribed.

Dry Powder Inhalers

DPIs are similar to MDIs, but they don't contain a propellant. Using a DPI requires inhaling more deeply and quickly to suck the medicine out of the device and into the lungs. DPIs are easy to use, as they don't require the coordination of taking a breath while actuating the device with your hand.

To use a DPI, simply place your mouth tightly over the mouthpiece and inhale quickly. A DPI inhaler should not be shaken before use (like an MDI), nor is a spacer needed.

Nebulizers

Inhaled medications like bronchodilators and corticosteroids can also be delivered via a nebulizer. A nebulizer is a machine that turns the liquid form of a drug into a fine mist that is then inhaled through a mouthpiece or facemask. Nebulizers are often used for treating very young children who have asthma. They are also used for older children and adults who have more severe lung disease, or who have difficulty using MDIs or dry powder inhalers.

The long-acting bronchodilator formoterol is available for use in a nebulizer. This drug is an alternative to MDI and DPI inhalers for COPD patients who may have difficulty using inhaler devices easily or correctly.

Treatment Options for COPD

Almost every person with COPD will be prescribed a short-acting bronchodilator (either a beta-agonist, an anticholinergic, or a combination of both) to use as needed to relieve shortness of breath, coughing, wheezing, and other symptoms. Some people will also need a long-acting bronchodilator and/or an anti-inflammatory drug. Your doctor will work with you to figure out the right drugs and combinations of drugs to relieve your symptoms.

For a person with mild COPD who has occasional symptoms, a short-acting bronchodilator alone may be sufficient to manage the condition. Two short-acting bronchodilators—a beta-agonist plus an anticholinergic—may also be prescribed. To simplify this regimen, a combination of a short-acting beta-agonist plus a short-acting anticholinergic is available in one inhaler (see Box 4-5, "Combination Drugs"). This may be the combination of albuterol plus ipratropium (Combivent Respimat, DuoNeb) or fenoterol plus ipratropium (Duovent).

As lung function deteriorates, additional medications will likely be necessary.

For people with moderate or severe COPD, who tend to experience symptoms more frequently, one or more long-acting bronchodilators will be added to the regimen. These drugs will be taken regularly every 12 or 24 hours. If acute episodes of breathlessness or coughing occur while taking these medications, a short-acting bronchodilator such as albuterol (Ventolin, Proventil, ProAir, VoSpire ER) can be used to quell the episodes.

For patients with more severe COPD, combinations of two long-acting bronchodilators are generally used. Combinations of two long-acting bronchodilators in a single inhaler are available.

Inhaled corticosteroids are recommended for people with moderate or severe COPD who do not get sufficient relief from bronchodilators, or who experience frequent exacerbations of symptoms. Inhaled corticosteroids have been shown to reduce flare-ups.

Some studies have found that use of inhaled corticosteroids, with or without a bronchodilator, increases the risk of developing pneumonia. Nevertheless, inhaled corticosteroids may decrease the risk of dying from pneumonia. Further research is needed to clarify these issues, and patients should discuss any concerns with their physician.

For people prescribed long-term use of both a long-acting bronchodilator and a corticosteroid, combinations of both in a single inhaler are available.

Roflumilast

Roflumilast (Daliresp) is a different type of drug for COPD. A PDE4 inhibitor, it works through a different mechanism than bronchodilators and anti-inflammatory drugs. Roflumilast is taken once a day to reduce inflammation in the lungs. It is not a bronchodilator.

Expectorants and Cough Suppressants

People with COPD often use expectorants, which can be obtained in cough medicines such as guaifenesin (Robitussin, Mucinex), to thin mucus and help to bring it up. However, there is little evidence to show that these medicines are helpful for people with COPD.

Cough suppressants should be avoided. Even though coughing can be bothersome, it has the important function of helping to clear mucus. This means that suppressing a cough may increase the risk of lung infection.

BOX 4-5

Combination Drugs	COPD	Asthma
Two short-term relief bronchodilators (beta-agonist plus anticholinergic)		
Combivent Respimat (albuterol plus ipratropium)	✓	
Duovent (fenoterol plus ipratropium)	✓	
Two longer-acting bronchodilators (beta-agonist plus anticholinergic)		
Anoro Ellipta (vilantero plus umeclidinium	✓	
Bevespi Aerosphere (formoterol fumarate plus glycopyrrolate)	✓	
Utibron Neohaler (indacaterol plus glycopyrrolate)	✓	
One bronchodilator (beta-agonist) plus one corticosteroid		
Advair Diskus (salmeterol plus fluticasone)	✓	✓
Symbicort (formoterol plus budesonide)	✓	✓
Dulera (formoterol plus mometasone)		✓
Breo Ellipta (vilanterol plus fluticasone)	✓	✓

Immunizations

For people with obstructive airway diseases, the flu can be very serious and even life threatening. The same applies to pneumonia, although this can be treated with antibiotics. Fortunately, vaccines are available to protect against influenza and some forms of pneumonia. It is extremely important that everyone with obstructive airway disease follow the recommended vaccination schedule, or their doctor's advice.

Flu Vaccine

People with COPD or other lung problems should receive an influenza vaccination once a year. The ideal time to get a flu shot is in October or November, as flu season runs from November to March.

Pneumococcal Vaccine

The pneumococcal vaccine protects against the bacteria that is the most common cause of pneumonia, *Streptococcus pneumoniae*. There are now two forms of pneumococcal vaccine, the Pneumovax and the Prevnar 13. It is recommended that all adults over age 65 receive a pneumococcal vaccination. Unlike the flu shot, which must be given every year in the fall, pneumococcal vaccination provides protection for at least five years. It can be given at any time of the year.

The pneumococcal vaccine is advised for all people with COPD age 65 and older. It also may be given to people with COPD who are younger than age 65 and have severe or very severe disease (FEV1 less than 40 percent of predicted), and recommended for people with asthma who are younger than age 65.

Treatment for Exacerbations

The most common cause of an exacerbation is a lung infection that may increase mucus production. In these cases, antibiotics may be used. Before prescribing an antibiotic, the doctor may send a sample of the sputum for analysis to determine whether the infection is bacterial or viral, since antibiotics are only effective against bacteria. Studies have shown that a short course (five days) of antibiotics is just as effective as taking antibiotics for longer than five days.

In 2017, the American Thoracic Society and European Respiratory Society issued joined guidelines on the management of COPD exacerbations. Their recommendations included:

- For ambulatory patients with an exacerbation of COPD, a short course of oral corticosteroids plus antibiotics.
- For patients hospitalized with an exacerbation, oral corticosteroids rather than intravenous corticosteroids, if possible.
- For patients hospitalized with an exacerbation causing respiratory failure, noninvasive mechanical ventilation.
- After being discharged for an exacerbation, pulmonary rehabilitation should begin within three weeks. It should not be started during hospitalization.

A recent study found that engaging in any amount of regular exercise following hospitalization for a COPD exacerbation actually reduces the risk of dying.

Alpha-1 Antitrypsin Therapy

Younger adults who inherited alpha-1 antitrypsin deficiency may be treated with alpha-1 antitrypsin augmentation therapy. This involves using a concentrated form of this protein that has been removed from donated blood and purified.

Augmentation therapy cannot reverse damage that has already been done to the lungs, but it can slow down any further decline in lung function. The therapy must be taken for life, and is very expensive. It must be administered by a healthcare professional in a doctor's office, hospital clinic, or home infusion service. The costs may be covered by private health insurance policies, but criteria for coverage can vary widely. Before beginning therapy, check with your insurance company. For people age 65 and older, Medicare covers at least part of the cost.

Pulmonary Rehabilitation

A very helpful addition to drug therapy for people at all stages of COPD is a specialized program called pulmonary rehabilitation. Pulmonary rehabilitation is a series of educational and structured exercises that enable people to make the most of their remaining lung capacity. People with COPD who engage in these programs have less shortness of breath, an increased ability to exercise, better quality of life, and less frequent hospitalizations than similar COPD patients who do not participate in pulmonary rehabilitation.

People with COPD tend to slow down their physical activity, since shortness of breath makes exertion increasingly difficult. Decreasing activity can start a vicious cycle of progressive deconditioning, and this leads to worsening of symptoms, more breathlessness, and less physical activity. Pulmonary rehabilitation is aimed at breaking that cycle.

A pulmonary rehabilitation program is more than an exercise program, although exercise is the most important component. In addition to exercise training, the program may include:

- Nutrition counseling
- Education about your condition
- Breathing strategies
- Energy-conserving techniques
- Help with smoking cessation
- Education about medications and how to take them

One study found that including music therapy in a pulmonary rehabilitation program provided added benefit. The participants, who attended six-week pulmonary rehab programs, also took part in weekly music therapy sessions that included playing wind instruments, and singing. They demonstrated greater improvements in symptoms such as shortness of breath, fatigue, and depression compared with COPD patients who had standard pulmonary rehab. Another study found that adding angiotensin-converting enzyme inhibitors (ACEI) might improve response to exercise training (see Box 4-6, "Common Medication Increases Exercise Capacity").

Most pulmonary rehabilitation programs last six weeks or longer. The exercises learned during the program should be continued at home once the program ends. Studies have found that pulmonary

NEW FINDING   BOX 4-6

Common Medication Increases Exercise Capacity

Angiotensin-converting enzyme (ACE) inhibitors, a common class of blood pressure-lowering drugs, have been shown to preserve muscle mass, strength, and walking speed. Researchers wondered whether the ACE inhibitor enalapril (Vasotec) might have a beneficial effect on patients undergoing pulmonary rehabilitation. They conducted a trial in which 80 patients with moderate-to-severe COPD undergoing pulmonary rehabilitation were randomized to enalapril or placebo. After 10 weeks, those in the ACE inhibitor group had significantly improved exercise capacity, compared with those taking placebo.

American Journal of Respiratory and Critical Care Medicine, December 1, 2016

Longer Pulmonary Rehabilitation Extends Benefits

The benefits of pulmonary rehabilitation tend to disappear over time. Researchers wondered whether continuing the program longer (for three years) would allow its benefits to endure.

After completing a standard eight-week pulmonary rehab program, 143 patients with moderate-to-severe COPD were randomized to a standard monitoring program, a maintenance intervention group, or a control group. Three measures were assessed: the six-minute walk test distance (6MWD) health-related quality of life, and the BODE index (which measures body mass index, airflow obstruction, dyspnea, and exercise capacity). All patients who had completed pulmonary rehabilitation showed significant improvements. Over the subsequent three years, those in the maintenance intervention group experienced a slight increase in 6MWD for one year, compared with the standard monitoring group. The BODE index score was maintained for two years. However, the improvements vanished after year two.

American Journal of Respiratory and Critical Care Medicine, March 1, 2017

rehabilitation benefits are generally sustained after the program ends, especially if the exercise training is maintained (see Box 4-7, "Longer Pulmonary Rehabilitation Extends Benefits").

One study found that people in the earlier derived greater benefits than those in the later stages. Although patients with less-advanced COPD had better results, those with severe COPD had improved ability to exercise and less shortness of breath. This research suggests that when it comes to pulmonary rehabilitation, the earlier it is done the better. However, patients with any stage of COPD can benefit from the program.

There are many pulmonary rehabilitation programs around the country. Your physician can most likely refer you to one; alternately, contact the American Lung Association or the American Association for Cardiovascular and Pulmonary Rehabilitation, which has a searchable online directory of pulmonary rehabilitation programs (see Appendix II: Resources). Be sure to ask your insurance carrier whether it covers pulmonary rehabilitation. Medicare coverage varies from state to state, so check with your physician or pulmonary rehabilitation provider to obtain the guidelines in your state.

Oxygen Therapy

People with severe COPD may have low levels of oxygen in their blood (a condition called hypoxemia). This may cause increased difficulty breathing, and further impair the ability to exercise. Low oxygen levels may also cause fatigue, memory loss, morning headaches, depression, and confusion. Over time, chronically low oxygen levels also can cause heart failure. Oxygen therapy can ensure the delivery of adequate oxygen to preserve the function of vital organs.

Many people with COPD have few, if any, symptoms that can be specifically linked to hypoxemia. To determine whether someone has hypoxemia, a physician will perform either an arterial blood gas test or pulse oximetry. In pulse oximetry, a noninvasive probe is attached to the finger, ear, or forehead to measure the amount of oxygen in the blood. The test may be done both at rest and while walking, since the oxygen level in the blood is often only low during activity.

Oxygen therapy usually is given only to people with very severe (stage IV) COPD (see Box 3-1, "Stages of COPD," in Chapter 3). In stage IV COPD, airflow is severely limited, and the amount of air that can be blown out in one second (FEV1) is less than 30 percent of what would be expected in someone without lung disease. For these people, long-term use of supplemental oxygen for more than 15 hours each day can prolong life and improve quality of life. Oxygen therapy can reduce shortness of breath during exertion, which makes it easier to perform basic daily activities. Oxygen therapy also may improve mental functioning, reduce depression, and help the heart.

The normal air we breathe contains about 21 percent oxygen. Providing more pure oxygen can increase the amount of oxygen taken into the lungs. The physician will prescribe a specific amount of supplemental oxygen, and provide instructions on when and how long it should be used, as well as which delivery method will be used. Supplemental oxygen may be used continuously (24 hours) or periodically, such as only during exercise or overnight. There are three methods for delivering oxygen, as explained below. With each system, the oxygen is breathed in through a mask or a nasal tube (cannula).

Compressed Oxygen Gas

Compressed oxygen gas is contained in tanks or cylinders of varying sizes. Large stationary tanks are used inside the home, while smaller, more portable tanks can be used on trips outside the home (they usually contain enough oxygen to last a few hours).

Liquid Oxygen

Cooling oxygen gas creates a liquid form of oxygen. When the liquid is warmed, it turns back into a gas that can be inhaled. Like compressed oxygen gas, liquid oxygen systems include a large tank for use in the home, and a small portable canister for use outside the home. This canister is filled with liquid oxygen from the indoor tank. One disadvantage of liquid oxygen systems is the tendency for the liquid to evaporate over time.

Oxygen Concentrator

An oxygen concentrator is an electric device that takes air from the room and separates the oxygen from other gases. The oxygen is then made available for inhaling through a mask or nasal cannula. This system does not require tanks of liquid or gaseous oxygen to be continuously refilled. The supply of oxygen is unlimited, and the device is small enough to be moved from room to room. Most oxygen concentrators require a continuous electrical source, and must be plugged into an electrical outlet. However there are portable oxygen concentrators that operate on battery power and may be used for exercise or travel.

Surgery
Lung Volume Reduction

Selected patients with advanced COPD may be candidates for a surgical procedure that can ease the effort of breathing and make walking and other daily activities more feasible. In this procedure, called lung volume reduction surgery, the parts of the lung that are most heavily damaged are removed.

As described previously, the destruction of alveoli in emphysema causes air to get trapped in the lungs. As a result, the lungs become enlarged (hyperinflated). Enlarged lungs can crowd the chest cavity and flatten the diaphragm, making it more difficult to breathe. Removing the hyperinflated portions of the lungs has the effect of improving lung function and quality of life.

The surgery doesn't cure emphysema, but it helps to relieve symptoms and may prolong life in some patients. However, the surgery is only effective in a minority of patients with emphysema. For this reason, it is very important that patients who are considering lung volume reduction surgery are carefully evaluated by a surgeon with experience in this highly specialized procedure.

Historically, lung volume reduction surgery involved opening the chest with an incision through the breastbone to gain access to the lungs. Today, it is more often done with several small incisions on both sides of the chest. A thin tube with a video camera on the end is inserted through one of the incisions. This allows the surgeon to see inside the body on a video monitor. Surgical instruments are inserted through the other incisions to remove the hyperinflated lung. Regardless of the procedure used, the operation requires hospital stay of five to 10 days.

Due to the risks of surgery, there is interest in trying to develop lung volume reduction techniques using bronchoscopy, a procedure that allows the doctor to view the airways through a thin instrument called a bronchoscope. At this time, the technique is considered experimental and is not available outside of research studies.

Medicare covers traditional lung volume reduction surgery for people who meet certain criteria, and requires that anyone contemplating the surgery first complete a certified pulmonary rehabilitation program.

Lung Transplantation

Lung transplantation may be considered for people with severe COPD who are otherwise healthy. This procedure is generally reserved for people with end-stage lung disease, but no other significant health problems. The criteria generally include an FEV1 of less than 20 percent of what would be predicted in someone without lung disease, as well as very low oxygen levels or very high carbon dioxide levels.

For patients with emphysema, either one or both lungs may be transplanted. The procedure generally results in improved lung function and better quality of life. However, there are risks involved in the surgery, and lung transplant recipients must take drugs to suppress their immune system for the remainder of their lives. These drugs are necessary to prevent the body from rejecting the new organ.

Smoking Cessation

Quitting smoking is an essential step for preventing and treating COPD. But as anyone who has quit smoking or tried to quit smoking can attest, it not so easy to accomplish. People with obstructive lung disease have a powerful incentive to quit smoking, yet many continue to light up. A study from the Centers of Disease Control and Prevention found that 46 percent of adults age 40 and older who have asthma or COPD still smoke.

Cigarette smoking is a powerful addiction, and simply knowing the laundry list of its effects is rarely enough to make smokers quit the habit. About 70 percent of adult smokers report that they want to quit completely, but very few people succeed in permanently quitting on their first attempt. First and foremost, quitting smoking requires motivation. It also requires understanding what you're up against, and getting the right type of help.

Nicotine Addiction

Nicotine is an addictive substance that acts on regions of the brain that produce pleasurable effects. Nicotine is carried in cigarette smoke into the lungs, where it is absorbed from the alveoli into the bloodstream. From there, it reaches the brain within about seven seconds and binds to receptors called nicotinic acetylcholine receptors, resulting in a release of brain chemicals called neurotransmitters. The primary neurotransmitter released from intake of nicotine is dopamine, which is believed to be linked to the region of the brain responsible for pleasurable feelings. Other neurotransmitters released when nicotine binds to nicotinic receptors also produce effects that reinforce tobacco use. These include stimulation, arousal, improved memory and attention, reduced stress, relaxation, improved mood, faster reaction time, and appetite suppression. Many smokers come to depend on smoking to produce these effects. However, because nicotine levels don't stay elevated in the blood for very long, the effects are short-lived and more cigarettes are needed to achieve them.

Upon quitting, many smokers report withdrawal symptoms, such as depressed mood, insomnia, irritability, frustration, anger, anxiety, difficulty concentrating, restlessness, decreased heart rate, and increased appetite or weight gain. These are relieved with smoking, making it especially difficult to quit.

The physiologic addiction to nicotine is only part of the story: There also is a large psychological and behavioral component. Smoking becomes a habit, and as such, smokers often associate smoking with certain activities or moods. For example, some people smoke a cigarette after a meal or with a drink, when they feel stressed, or to perk themselves up when they feel down. Smokers also come to associate the pleasurable effects of smoking with the ritual of smoking. They may enjoy just holding a cigarette, the act of lighting it, or the smell and taste of the smoke.

Getting Help to Quit

Because smoking is associated with physiological, behavioral, and psychological factors, all three must be addressed when attempting to quit. Studies have shown that some combination of counseling, social support, and pharmacologic therapies usually is necessary. It usually takes more than one try to quit for good—the average is seven attempts—but the benefits are worth it.

It all starts with the decision to quit. Guidelines published by the Agency for Healthcare Research and Quality recommend beginning by setting a firm quit date, preferably within two weeks. Some helpful strategies for quitting can be found in Box 4-8, "Strategies to Quit Smoking." Enlisting the support of family and friends is essential. Some form of counseling—either an individual or group counseling program—is advised. Internet-based chat rooms can also be helpful. Quit lines have been set up in many states (www.smokefree.gov; 1-800-QUITNOW) to connect smokers to relevant resources. Some smokers have been helped to quit with acupuncture or hypnosis. For people age 65 and older, who smoke and have a disease or adverse health effects linked to tobacco use, Medicare Part B will cover smoking cessation counseling. Two smoking cessation attempts are allowed each year, and for each attempt, Medicare will pay for up to four counseling sessions.

Breaking the smoking habit will most likely require coming up with new problem-solving and stress-reducing techniques to replace

BOX 4-8

Strategies to Quit Smoking

- Set a date to quit.
- Resolve to quit "cold turkey," rather than gradually cutting back.
- Remove all cigarettes and ashtrays from your home, car, and place of work.
- Tell family and friends you intend quitting, and ask for their support.
- Use some form of nicotine replacement (patch, gum, or lozenge).
- Talk to your doctor about medications that may help you.
- Call 1-800-QUIT NOW (1-800-784-8669) to find the quitline in your state.
- Find counseling (individual, group, or telephone) that you are comfortable with.
- If you don't succeed the first time, try again.

smoking. For example, it can be helpful to identify situations or activities that increase your risk for smoking, and discuss new types of coping skills with a counselor or fellow smokers who are quitting. Also try to minimize time spent with smokers, to reduce temptation.

Medications That Can Help You Quit

Several types of pharmacologic therapies are available to relieve nicotine withdrawal symptoms:

Nicotine Replacement Therapies

These are available in skin patches, gums, lozenges, inhalers, and as a nasal spray. The patch, gum, and lozenges can be obtained without a prescription. Nicotine gum is not chewed like regular gum—in order for the nicotine to be absorbed, the gum must be chewed a few times, and then held between the cheek and gum.

The nicotine patch maintains a steady blood level of nicotine. This avoids the ups and downs of nicotine levels during smoking, and disrupts the "crave-and-reward" cycle. A step-down program is usually recommended when using the nicotine patch. This program starts with a higher dose of 21 milligrams (mg) per day, which is reduced to a moderate dose (14 mg/day), and finally a low dose (7 mg/day).

E-cigarettes contain nicotine, and some smokers switch to these vapor-producing devices to help them quit tobacco cigarettes. The effectiveness of nicotine replacement therapies such as the gum and patch are established. E-cigarettes are still being studied as an aid to quitting, and two questions remain unanswered: First, are e-cigarettes safe? Second, are they an effective tool for quitting? One study found that smokers who used e-cigarettes were actually less likely to quit smoking than those who never used them.

Bupropion (Zyban)

Bupropion (Zyban), which requires a doctor's prescription, has been shown to help eliminate withdrawal symptoms. It appears that the drug works best when used in conjunction with one of the nicotine replacement therapies.

Varenicline (Chantix)

This is another drug available by prescription only. Varenicline works by binding to some of the nicotinic receptors, thereby blocking nicotine from binding to these receptors. This results in a reduction in the craving for nicotine, and decreases the pleasurable effects of smoking. Studies have shown the drug to be generally effective at helping people to quit smoking. However, some people who take the drug experience dramatic changes in mood and behavior. The manufacturer advises stopping the drug and contacting a healthcare provider immediately if agitation, depressed mood, changes in behavior, or suicidal thoughts or behavior occur. Some people who use varenicline have a decreased tolerance to alcohol, and get drunk more easily—therefore, people who use the drug are advised to decrease the amount of alcohol they consume.

There are numerous resources to help people quit smoking. Some of these are listed in the "Appendix II: Resources" section. If you try and fail, don't be discouraged: You are not alone. Perhaps you just need to try a different technique until you find one that works for you.

Health Benefits of Smoking Cessation

Some of the benefits of quitting occur relatively quickly, while others can take 10 or more years (see Box 4-9, "Timeline for Health Benefits After Smoking Cessation"). Soon after quitting, blood circulation and lung function begin to improve. Within one to two years, the risk for heart disease decreases. The risk for developing cancer declines with the number of years of smoking cessation.

A large study of more than 104,000 women quantified some of the risk reduction with smoking cessation:

- Those who quit smoking had a 13 percent lower risk of dying from any cause within the first five years of quitting, compared with women who continued to smoke.
- The excess risk of death from any cause reached the level of never-smokers 20 years after quitting.
- Much of the reduction in the risk of dying from heart disease was realized within the first five years.
- Five to 10 years after quitting, death from any type of lung disease was reduced by 18 percent. After 20 years, it reached the level of never-smokers.
- About 64 percent of deaths among current smokers and 28 percent of deaths among former smokers were attributable to cigarette smoking.
- Lung cancer mortality was reduced 21 percent within five years of smoking cessation. It took 30 years to completely eliminate the excess risk.

Lifestyle Tips to Maintain Lung Function

In addition to quitting smoking and taking prescribed medications, people with COPD can take steps to improve their health and possibly slow down the damage caused by the disease. Strategies include eating a healthy diet, exercising regularly, learning special breathing techniques, and making changes in day-to-day life, among others. Even staying cool can have important benefits: One study found that high indoor and outdoor temperatures were linked to more symptoms. Being in hot indoor environments also worsened lung function.

Healthy habits are recommended for everyone, but are especially necessary for those with chronic lung disease.

Eat Right

Your body needs the energy provided by food to function, and that includes breathing. In fact, oxygen is a necessary part of the process of breaking down food into energy (called metabolism). Energy, in turn, is needed for the process of breathing. For people with COPD, difficulty breathing may make it difficult to eat properly, creating a downward cycle that can lead to malnourishment and even greater breathing problems.

BOX 4-9

Timeline for Health Benefits After Smoking Cessation

Within 20 minutes of quitting smoking your body begins a series of changes that continue for years:

- **20 minutes:** Your heart rate drops.
- **12 hours:** The carbon monoxide level in your blood drops to normal.
- **Two weeks to three months:** Your heart attack risk begins to drop, and your lung function begins to improve.
- **One to nine months:** Your coughing and shortness of breath decrease.
- **One year:** Your added risk of coronary heart disease is half that of a smoker's.
- **Five years:** Your stroke risk is reduced to that of a nonsmoker's five to 15 years after quitting.
- **10 years:** Your lung cancer death rate is about half that of a smoker's. Your risk for cancers of the mouth, throat, esophagus, bladder, kidney, and pancreas decreases.
- **15 years:** Your risk of coronary heart disease is back to that of a nonsmoker.

BOX 4-10

Calories Needed Each Day

The number of calories you need each day depends on your sex, age, and level of activity. This table shows about how many calories people of average weight should consume each day to maintain their weight.

	AGE	RELATIVELY SEDENTARY	MODERATELY ACTIVE	ACTIVE
WOMEN	31-50	1,800	2,000	2,200
	51+	1,600	1,800	2,000–2,200
MEN	31–40	2,400	2,600	2,800–3,000
	41–60	2,200	2,400–2,600	2,800
	61+	2,000	2,200–2,400	2,400–2,600

Dietary Guidelines for Americans, 2015-2020

About one-third of people with COPD are malnourished, and experience weight loss. Malnutrition can worsen lung function and also compromise the immune system. A compromised immune system can render a person with COPD susceptible to infections and other illnesses.

It is extremely important for people with COPD to consume the recommended number of calories, and try to maintain a healthy weight. If you are underweight, it means your body has fewer stores of energy to draw from. Being overweight also can be problematic, since carrying extra weight means the heart has to work harder, which makes breathing more difficult.

A well-balanced diet that provides an adequate number of calories is necessary for good health. The recommended caloric intake varies by age and level of activity (see Box 4-10, "Calories Needed Each Day").

Keep in mind that people with COPD expend extra energy in the simple act of breathing. For a person with COPD, the act of breathing may burn 10 times as many calories as it does for someone without lung disease. This means that even more calories may be required to maintain proper weight.

Foods to Prioritize

The source of calories is important. The U.S. Department of Agriculture (USDA) has established sound nutrition guidelines, which are available at www.choosemyplate.gov. You might also consider consulting a registered dietitian who specializes in COPD and can work with you to develop an individualized food plan.

The USDA recommends consuming foods and beverages that are rich in nutrients and come from the basic food groups. Try to avoid foods with little nutritional value that supply only empty calories, as this can cause you to become obese, yet malnourished (see Box 4-11, "Obesity Detrimental to Patients With COPD"). Your diet should emphasize fruits, vegetables, whole grains, and dairy products. The diet should also include protein from lean meats, poultry, and fish, along with beans, eggs, and nuts. Try to limit your consumption of saturated fats, trans fats, cholesterol, salt (sodium), and sugar. Sodium is particularly problematic because it can cause fluid retention, which can interfere with breathing.

One study found that people with COPD who ate a healthy diet that included fish, grapefruit, bananas, and cheese had better lung function and fewer symptoms than those who did not eat these foods. The researchers noted that these particular foods may not by themselves be the key to improved health—rather, eating them indicates the person most likely eats an overall healthy diet that includes fish, fruit, and dairy products.

NEW FINDING BOX 4-11

Obesity Detrimental to People With COPD

Just as being underweight is dangerous for people with COPD, being obese can be harmful too. Researchers looked at the body weight of 3,631 participants in a multicenter study of patients with COPD, and found that the number of comorbidities increased along with obesity class. The more obese the patients, the greater the likelihood they would have more difficulty breathing and walking. Their risk for exacerbations also increased. All of these factors led to a poorer quality of life.

Chest, January 15, 2017

Foods to Avoid

Avoid foods that cause gas or bloating, as this can make breathing more difficult. Gas-producing foods include broccoli, cauliflower, beans, and carbonated beverages.

Other Diet Tips

Drink plenty of fluids, which help to thin mucus and make it easier to cough up. Try for six to eight glasses (eight fluid ounces each) per day. Water, milk, and fruit juice are the best sources, but coffee, tea, and soft drinks also count. Alcoholic beverages, such as wine and beer, contribute to fluid intake, but should be consumed only in limited amounts.

If breathing problems make eating difficult, try eating four to six small meals a day, rather than three large ones. You might also try eating the largest meal early in the day, so that you have more energy for the rest of the day. Take your time preparing meals, and choose foods that are easy to prepare. You don't want to expend too much energy making a meal, only to have little energy left to eat it. Eat slowly, in a relaxed setting. Digestion requires energy, so wait an hour or more after eating before engaging in activities.

Exercise Regularly

People in all stages of COPD experience a decline in their ability to engage in physical activity as the disease worsens. Although it may seem difficult to exercise when breathing is a problem, regular exercise can actually improve lung function. It also keeps muscles strong, and improves overall health. A recent study of people with COPD found that those who got no exercise at all were less able to be physically active and had weaker muscle strength compared with people who were at least somewhat physically active.

If you feel daunted by the idea of exercising, keep in mind that the level of exertion required is relative to your health and ability. You don't need to be an athlete to benefit from exercise—in fact, you should begin by having a discussion with your doctor to determine the most appropriate type of exercise and level of intensity.

If you've been in a pulmonary rehabilitation program, continue the exercises on your own after finishing the program. If you haven't been in one of these programs, be sure to increase your physical activity slowly from your present level. Walking and swimming are good ways to get exercise without overexerting yourself. Try to walk a little farther and for longer periods each day. Try to work up to 20 to 30 minutes of physical activity three to five times a week. The key is to do it on a regular basis (daily, or at least several times each week). Research has shown that increasing physical activity decreases hospitalizations due to exacerbations of COPD. One study found that people with COPD who engaged in any regular exercise were about one-third less likely to be readmitted to the hospital within 30 days of being discharged. The benefit was greatest for those who exercised 150 minutes or more a week.

Before beginning an exercise, warm up your muscles by doing some stretches. If walking is your chosen activity, start at a slow pace and gradually walk faster. It may help to walk or exercise with friends,

BOX 4-12

BOX 4-13

Pursed-Lip Breathing

- Sit comfortably, with your feet on the floor, and relax.

- Breathe in through your nose.

- Breathe out slowly and evenly through pursed lips. To purse your lips, position them as though you are about to whistle (lips mostly closed, with a small opening in the center). Breathing out should take twice as long as inhaling.

- Repeat the technique several times until shortness of breath diminishes.

Diaphragmatic Breathing

- Lie comfortably on your back.

- Place one hand on your upper chest and one on your stomach.

- Breathe normally for a minute, and notice whether your chest or stomach rises with each intake of breath. If your chest expands, try to focus on breathing with your diaphragm (which would cause your stomach to rise).

- Inhale slowly through your nose.

- Slowly exhale through pursed lips.

- Rest and repeat. Continue for five to 10 minutes.

making it a social occasion. Be sure to go at your own pace, and don't compare yourself to anyone else. Keep a diary to record your exercise goals and track your progress.

Control Your Breathing

Breathing techniques, such as pursed-lip breathing and diaphragmatic breathing, can help to make the most of every breath you take. Talk to your physician or respiratory therapist about these techniques to find out if they might be useful for you.

Air that gets trapped in the lungs can cause shortness of breath. Air trapping can occur from breathing too fast, or because airways are narrowed, and alveoli are damaged. Pursed-lip breathing slows the pace of breathing and increases air pressure in the lungs, which helps the airways stay open. If you feel short of breath from exertion, stop for a few minutes and practice pursed-lip breathing to get fresh air flowing into your lungs (see Box 4-12, "Pursed-Lip Breathing").

Diaphragmatic breathing facilitates deeper breathing. The diaphragm is a dome-shaped muscle in the abdomen that is involved in the mechanical process of breathing. In people with COPD, the diaphragm and other muscles involved in breathing can weaken. Using a diaphragmatic breathing technique (see Box 4-13, "Diaphragmatic Breathing") can help to strengthen these muscles, slow down your breathing rate, increase your blood oxygen levels, and allow you to use less effort to breathe.

Breathe Clean Air

Keep the air in your home as clear of irritants as possible. For example:
- Don't smoke, and don't allow anyone else to smoke in the house.
- Keep all fumes and strong smells out. This includes air fresheners, scented candles, and fragrant cleaning products.
- If you must have painting done, stay out of the house until it is finished.
- Avoid smoke from wood fires.

Travel Comfortably

Having a chronic lung disease such as COPD may require making special arrangements for traveling, particularly by airplane. Those who require oxygen therapy will first need to obtain permission from their physician to fly. They must also notify the airline in advance of travel to arrange for using oxygen during the flight.

Some people who don't require oxygen therapy at home may need supplemental oxygen while flying. This is because the air pressure inside an airplane cabin is lower than it is on the ground, especially when the airplane is taking off and landing. Low air pressure decreases the amount of oxygen in the air. People without lung disease can adapt to the changes in air pressure, but for a person with severe COPD, even a small change in air pressure may cause an exacerbation of symptoms.

Always discuss air travel plans with your physician. Blood oxygen measurements will likely be needed to determine whether supplemental oxygen will be required. The doctor will also need to provide a letter to the airline. During the flight, the oxygen will be provided by the airline (likely at a fee). Passengers are not allowed to bring their own liquid or gas oxygen canisters on board an airplane. However, some airlines allow patients to use their own portable concentrators during flights. Empty cylinders and equipment likely are allowed only as checked baggage.

Information about which airlines allow use of oxygen on flights, along with their policies, is available from the Airline Oxygen Council of America (see Appendix II: Resources).

Relax and Take Care of Yourself

Anxiety, stress, and fatigue are common in everyday life and can lead to health problems even for otherwise healthy people. For people with COPD they can exacerbate the condition, leading to worsened lung function, infections, and other health problems (see Box 4-14, "Know Your Limits").

Coping with COPD may feel overwhelming at times. Sharing feelings and concerns with loved ones and asking for their help may ease some of the burden. Joining a support group for people with COPD may be even more helpful. The American Lung Association (see Appendix II: Resources) is a good resource for finding a local support group.

BOX 4-14

Know Your Limits

Having a chronic health condition requires that you take very good care of yourself. This means knowing your limits.

- Rest when you are tired.
- Take the time you need for everyday tasks.
- Wear clothes that are easy to put on and take off.
- Avoid situations that might be stressful.
- Stay away from crowds during flu season, and from people you know to have a cold or the flu.
- Keep phone numbers for your doctor, hospital, and important contact people in an easily accessible place.
- Keep and continually update a list of all the medications you are taking. Put it someplace accessible, so it can easily be taken to the hospital or any doctor's appointment.

ASTHMA

BOX 5-1

Asthma Attack

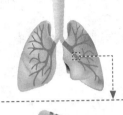

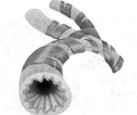

Airways before an
asthma attack.

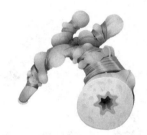

In an asthma attack, airways fill with
mucus and swell, and the muscles
around the airway contract.

Asthma is a chronic disease that often starts in childhood but can occur for the first time in adulthood, even later in life. According to the Centers for Disease Control and Prevention (CDC), 18.4 million adults and 6.2 million children in the United States have asthma.

Asthma causes inflammation in the airways, producing episodes of coughing, wheezing, breathlessness, and chest tightness. Inflammation also causes the airways to secrete excess mucus, which clogs the airway, restricting the flow of air. In addition, the muscles surrounding the airways sometimes suddenly contract, causing the airway to narrow (see Box 5-1, "Asthma Attack").

Asthma attacks usually occur in response to a specific trigger, such as pollen, house-dust mites, animal dander (shed skin flakes), or mold, all of which can also cause allergies. One study found that about 75 percent of 20 to 40 year olds with asthma, and 65 percent of adults aged 55 and older with asthma, have at least one allergy. Exposure to cold air, exercise, a viral infection, airborne irritants (chemicals, tobacco, or wood smoke), stress, or strong emotions can also spark an asthma attack.

For most people with asthma, airway narrowing is reversible. The airway will return to normal spontaneously or with the aid of a bronchodilator drug. In some people with long-standing or severe asthma, however, the constant inflammation causes permanent changes to the airways. For these people, the condition may not be completely reversible, even with medication (see Box 5-2, "Exacerbation-Prone Asthma May Be a Distinct Phenotype"). It is often very difficult or impossible to distinguish this form of asthma from COPD—consequently, the treatment of severe persistent asthma and COPD often closely resemble each other.

Asthma is on the increase among children younger than 18, and it is more common in boys than girls. Women are more prone to adult-onset asthma than men, and more adult women than adult men have asthma. It can first appear in older age. The diagnosis of asthma in older adults may be missed because other health problems with similar symptoms (such as heart disease or COPD) may coexist.

What Causes Asthma?

The exact cause of asthma is not fully known, but it is believed to result from a combination of genetic and environmental factors. In other words, some people inherit genes that make them susceptible to developing asthma. Numerous genes have been identified that appear to play some role in asthma. When people with these genes are exposed to environmental factors during a crucial time in their development, their immune system is altered in a way that produces chronic inflammation in the airways and sensitivity to certain stimuli. This leads to asthma attacks.

Immunity Gone Awry

Inflammation is part of the normal protective response of the body's immune system. The highly complex immune system defends the body against harmful substances such as bacteria, viruses, and irritants that can enter through any opening, such as the mouth, the nostrils, or a wound. The immune system generates inflammation for a variety of reasons, including to serve as a barrier against the spread of infection, and to promote healing.

Normally, inflammation subsides after the harmful invader has been eliminated. But sometimes, inflammation becomes chronic and can be problematic, as happens in people with asthma.

The immune system is not static. It is continuously responding and evolving based on what the body encounters from the external environment, which can include bacteria, viruses, and pollutants, among other things. It also responds to internal factors, such as stress.

One theory is that for asthma to develop, very specific combinations of genes and environmental factors must be present. Environmental exposures that have been most clearly linked to the development of asthma are airborne allergens and viral respiratory infections (such as pneumonia, a cold, or flu). One study found that children who had a lung infection such as pneumonia before age three had nearly double the risk of asthma or wheezing later on.

Smoking

One study suggests that cigarette smoking may increase the risk for developing asthma. In addition, cigarette smoking during pregnancy has been linked to a greater risk for the child to experience bouts of wheezing, although it is not certain that this leads to asthma.

Air Pollution (Particularly High Ozone Levels)

Some research suggests that young children exposed to traffic-related pollution are more likely to develop respiratory problems, such as wheezing. Some evidence suggests that babies born to women exposed to air pollution during pregnancy may be at greater risk for asthma.

Obesity

The CDC recently reported that more overweight and obese adults have asthma than adults of normal weight. As obesity rates in the U.S. have climbed, so have asthma rates. About 7 percent of normal-weight people have asthma, compared with 11 percent of obese adults, and 15 percent of obese women. The reason for the connection is unknown.

Interestingly, underweight women also have an increased risk for asthma, and both obese and underweight women who drink and smoke have twice the risk for asthma compared with women of normal weight who don't drink or smoke.

Gaining control of asthma is more difficult for obese patients than for those with normal body weight. Recent research suggests exercise may help (see Box 5-3, "Exercise Helps Obese Asthma Patients Gain Control.")

Stress

Several studies have found that children who suffer adversity, such as physical abuse, the death of a parent, divorced or separated parents, or living with someone who has a drug or alcohol problem,

NEW FINDING BOX 5-2

Exacerbation-Prone Asthma May Be a Distinct Phenotype

Why are some patients with asthma prone to exacerbations, while others are not? That's a key question researchers sought to answer. They examined patients in the National Heart, Lung, and Blood Institute's Severe Asthma Research Program-3, and noted the number of exacerbations they had in the past year: none, one or two, three or more. Of the 709 patients, 41 percent had no exacerbations and 24 percent had three or more. Those who were exacerbation-prone did not exhibit the factors associated with asthma severity. However, bronchodilator responsiveness, blood eosinophil level, and body mass index were associated with more frequent exacerbations, as were chronic sinusitis and gastroesophageal reflux. The researchers concluded that exacerbation-prone asthma may be a distinct phenotype from typical asthma.

American Journal of Respiratory and Critical Care Medicine, February 1, 2017

NEW FINDING BOX 5-3

Exercise Helps Obese Asthma Patients Gain Control

It is difficult for many obese patients with asthma to gain control over their disease. Bariatric surgery can help, but so can exercise, researchers have found. Fifty-five obese patients with asthma were assigned to a weight-loss program that did or did not include exercise. The program that included exercise incorporated both aerobic and muscle-strengthening training. The program that did not include exercise incorporated breathing and stretching exercises, along with psychological therapy. In three months, those who exercised lost more weight, gained aerobic capacity, and saw improvements in lung function, anti-inflammatory biomarkers, vitamin D levels, and airway and systemic inflation. In other words, they gained better control over their asthma than those who did not exercise.

American Journal of Respiratory and Critical Care Medicine, January 1, 2017

mental illness, or has served time in jail, are at increased risk of developing asthma. The reason for this association is not known, but it is possible that childhood adversity causes chronic stress, which can lead to asthma.

Mold Exposure

A few studies have found that infants who live in homes with mold are more likely to develop asthma than those who are not exposed to mold.

Anemia

One study found that the children of women who had anemia during pregnancy are at increased risk for asthma.

Birth Country

Simply being born in the U.S. appears to increase the risk for asthma. Children and teenagers who are born in other countries and immigrate to the U.S. are about half as likely to have asthma and allergies as children born in the U.S., according to one study. The "Westernization Theory" may be responsible. This theory postulates that an exceptionally clean environment in childhood may prevent a child's immune system from fully developing. Such children are more likely to have asthma and allergies than children raised in countries where less-sanitary living standards are the norm. However, it is also possible that children from Western backgrounds see physicians more frequently, and have common medical conditions such as asthma recognized earlier in life. This leads to more diagnoses, which may account in part for why asthma seems more common in industrialized countries.

Breastfeeding

Some studies have found that breastfeeding may help protect children from asthma, but the reason for a potential link between breastfeeding and better lung function is not known. The World Health Organization recommends breastfeeding exclusively for the first six months of life.

Symptoms of Asthma

The most common symptom of asthma is a cough, although wheezing (a high-pitched whistling sound, especially when exhaling), chest tightness, and shortness of breath also are common.

In people with asthma, respiratory symptoms worsen in response to particular stimuli. The symptoms may occur, and often seem to worsen, at night. In some people, especially young children, the only symptom of asthma will be a cough that is worse at night.

More than one-third of adults with asthma suffer from insomnia, and, as a result, are sleepy during the daytime. This can lead to depression, anxiety, and diminished quality of life.

An asthma attack may occur suddenly or may begin slowly, with gradually worsening symptoms. It may end quickly or last for several hours. In some cases, an initial asthma attack will ease up but then be followed by a second, possibly more severe, attack. Some severe asthma attacks will cause significant difficulty breathing, and the lips and fingernails may assume a gray or blue tinge from lack of oxygen (cyanosis). In the event of a severe asthma attack, it may be necessary to call Emergency Services (911) or go to a hospital emergency room or a physician's office for immediate treatment.

Research suggests that people who are obese (a body mass index greater than 30) may experience worse asthma symptoms than those of normal weight, due to dynamic hyperinflation. This means that air that is breathed in gets trapped in the lungs and is not exhaled, and the result is a greater feeling of breathlessness.

Asthma Triggers

Pollen and Mold

Outdoor allergens include pollen and mold.

Allergy season, when pollen counts are highest, varies depending on where you live. To limit exposure to pollen and outdoor mold during allergy season, keep windows closed as much as possible and try to stay indoors around midday, when pollen and some mold spore counts are highest. It may be necessary to increase the dose of medication just before and during allergy season if you are sensitive to pollen and outdoor mold.

Indoor mold can grow wherever there is dampness or wetness. To keep the house as dry as possible, make sure faucets, pipes, and other sources of water are not leaking. Clean any surfaces that have mold. Basements, which can be damp, should be dehumidified if possible.

Pet Allergies

For people who have an allergic response to cats, dogs, or other animals with fur, it is the animals' flakes of skin (dander) or dried saliva that cause the reaction. The best option for people with asthma triggered by animal dander is not to have a pet, or to have a hypoallergenic pet. For those who do not wish to deprive themselves of pet ownership, some precautions may help. The pet may be kept outdoors, or at minimum, out of the bedroom. Carpets can attract animal hair, dander, and dried saliva, so replace them with wood or tile floors, or keep the pet out of carpeted rooms.

Insects

Some people with asthma are allergic to the dried droppings and remains of cockroaches. To make your home as unappealing as possible to cockroaches, never leave food out, keep garbage in a closed container, and fix plumbing leaks. Use poison baits, powders, gels, or pastes to kill cockroaches if you see them.

Dust mites are microscopic bugs that can live in carpets, furniture, mattresses, and bedding. Dust mites are harmless to humans, but they can trigger allergies and asthma attacks. Strategies for avoiding dust mites are found in Box 5-4, "Avoiding Dust Mites."

Smoke, Strong Odors, and Sprays

Smoke from cigarettes, cigars, pipes, or a wood-burning stove or fireplace can trigger an asthma attack in some people. It is best to stay away from people who are smoking, and to keep your home smoke-free.

BOX 5-4

Avoiding Dust Mites

Dust mites are tiny "bugs" (relatives of the spider) you cannot see that live in cloth or carpet. Follow these steps to reduce their allergen effects:

- Encase your mattress in a special dust mite-proof cover.*

- Encase your pillow in a special dust mite-proof cover* or wash the pillow each week in hot water (the water must be hotter than 130°F to kill the mites, though cooler water also can be effective if detergent and bleach are used).

- Wash the sheets and blankets on your bed each week in hot water.

- Reduce indoor humidity to or below 60 percent (ideally 30 to 50 percent). Dehumidifiers or central air conditioners can do this.

- Try not to sleep or lie on cloth-covered cushions or furniture.

- Remove carpeting from your bedroom.

- Keep stuffed toys out of the bed, or wash the toys weekly in hot water (or cooler water with detergent and bleach). Placing toys weekly in a dryer or freezer may help. Prolonged exposure to dry heat or freezing can kill mites, but won't remove allergens.

*For more information on products, contact the Asthma and Allergy Foundation of America, or the American College of Allergy, Asthma, and Immunology (see Appendix II: Resources).

National Heart, Lung, and Blood Institute Guidelines for the Diagnosis and Management of Asthma

A person with asthma who smokes should quit, and should encourage other people living in the home who smoke to stop as well. Smoking increases the risk for numerous diseases, including cancer and heart disease, as well as COPD.

Strong odors and sprays, such as perfume, aftershave, scented body lotions, hair spray, talcum powder, paint, new carpet, and others can also be problematic for some people with asthma. Exposure to these irritants should be limited as much as possible.

Exercise

To minimize the chance of experiencing symptoms while exercising or engaging in sports, be sure to spend about 10 minutes warming up before engaging in vigorous exercise. Check the air quality and pollen levels if you are allergic to pollen, and try to exercise during times when air quality is good and pollen levels are low.

Many people with asthma also use their rescue inhaler 10 minutes prior to exercising, which decreases the chances of an attack during exercise and also improves exercise performance for many.

Medications

Some people with asthma are sensitive to certain medications. Drugs that can trigger asthma symptoms include beta-blockers (used to treat high blood pressure), aspirin, and nonsteroidal anti-inflammatory drugs (NSAIDs). NSAIDs are used for pain relief and include common over-the-counter drugs such as ibuprofen (Advil, Motrin) and naproxen (Aleve). Aspirin and NSAIDs trigger asthma symptoms in about 3 to 5 percent of adults with asthma.

For people who are bothered by any of these medications there are alternatives. Your physician can make specific recommendations.

Sulfites in Foods

Some foods and drinks contain sulfite compounds. These compounds work as a preservative to prevent discoloration, and can be found in beer, wine, processed potatoes, dried fruit, sauerkraut, and shrimp. About 5 percent of people with asthma have a worsening of symptoms when they eat foods containing sulfites. The only remedy for these individuals is to avoid sulfite-containing foods. Foods and beverages that contain sulfites must indicate this on the label.

Other Triggers

Some people find that viral infections, changes in weather, strong emotions, or their menstrual cycle worsen asthma symptoms, or even trigger an attack.

Diagnosing Asthma

A physician will suspect asthma in a person who has characteristic symptoms that recur and are triggered or worsened by certain stimuli, such as the triggers mentioned above.

To make the diagnosis, a physician will take a detailed medical history, conduct a physical examination that includes listening to the chest for wheezing sounds, and perform a spirometry test. This often involves bronchodilator reversibility testing to determine if the airflow obstruction is reversible, which is typical in asthma. The spirometry test also may be used to rule out other possible causes of symptoms, such as COPD. While taking a medical history, the physician is likely to ask the questions in Box 5-5, "Medical History Questions."

Treating Asthma

Asthma can't be cured, but it can be effectively managed by preventing asthma attacks as much as possible, and treating them when they occur. The goals of asthma treatment are to reduce the intensity and frequency of asthma attacks, and to prevent any adverse effects of asthma (such as the need for hospitalization), as well as any side effects of asthma medications. Ideally, if asthma is well managed:

- There will be few bothersome symptoms. This means that symptoms will occur in the daytime no more than twice each week, and symptoms in the night will be limited to no more than twice each month.
- Use of an inhaled bronchodilator will be needed only two or fewer times per week.
- Normal daily activities, such as work, school attendance, exercise, and participation in athletics, will not be hindered.
- Airflow, as measured with a peak flow meter, will be normal.
- The need for hospitalization or use of oral steroids for asthma symptoms will occur no more than once a year.

Achieving these goals involves eliminating or minimizing asthma triggers, and using appropriate drug therapy (usually inhaled beta-agonists and inhaled corticosteroids). For people with asthma that is triggered by allergies, immunotherapy (commonly known as allergy shots) may be used. Everyone with asthma should follow the recommended schedule for influenza and pneumonia vaccinations.

It is very important not to rely on treating asthma attacks, but to prevent them from occurring. This means identifying the substances or circumstances that trigger attacks and doing everything possible to avoid or limit exposure to them.

Drug Therapy for Asthma

The most important step in asthma is to avoid asthma triggers—this will prevent asthma attacks from occurring. However, most people with asthma will need medications.

There are two general types of asthma medications:

- Long-term control medications must be taken daily to prevent symptoms, generally by reducing inflammation. They will not provide quick relief for symptoms.
- Quick-relief medications are usually fast-acting bronchodilators that work by relaxing airway muscles, promptly relieving symptoms. They are used to open airways during an asthma attack or just before exposure to a known trigger, such as exercise.

For the most part, long-term control medications should keep

BOX 5-5

Medical History Questions

- Do the symptoms occur seasonally (for example, during pollen season) or year round?
- How often do the symptoms occur, and how long do they last?
- Do the symptoms tend to occur at a particular time of day (at night, early morning, etc.)?
- At what age did the symptoms begin?
- Are there any identifiable triggers for the symptoms?
- Have you had any viral respiratory infections?
- Is there anything about the home environment that could trigger asthma (for example, the age of the home, its location, the type of cooling and heating system it uses, the presence of a wood-burning stove, mold or mildew, or pets, among others)?
- Does anyone in the home smoke cigarettes?
- Do the symptoms change with exercise or exposure to cold air?
- Are the symptoms sparked by intense emotions, stress, drugs (such as aspirin, anti-inflammatory drugs, beta-blockers [used for treating hypertension] or others), or food additives (such as sulfites)?
- Do you have any other medical conditions that may cause or exacerbate the symptoms?
- Do any close relatives have asthma, allergy, sinusitis, eczema, or nasal polyps?

BOX 5-6

Intermittent Asthma

- Daytime asthma symptoms occur two or fewer days per week.

- Nighttime awakenings due to symptoms occur two or fewer times per month.

- The need for a bronchodilator (a short-acting beta-agonist) to relieve symptoms occurs fewer than two times per week.

- Between the times when symptoms are experienced, there is no interference with normal activities.

- FEV1, as measured by spirometry, is consistently normal (80 percent or more of predicted normal) during the times between active symptoms.

- The FEV1/FVC ratio is normal between active symptoms.

- Oral steroids are required to treat severe symptoms one or fewer times per year.

National Heart, Lung, and Blood Institute Guidelines for the Diagnosis and Management of Asthma

BOX 5-7

Mild Persistent Asthma

- Symptoms occur more than twice weekly, but less than daily.

- There are three to four nighttime awakenings per month due to asthma.

- Use of a bronchodilator (short-acting beta-agonist) to relieve symptoms is necessary more than two times a week, but not daily.

- There is minor interference with normal activities.

- FEV1, as measured by spirometry, is consistently normal (80 percent or more of predicted normal).

- The FEV1/FVC ratio is normal.

- Oral steroids are required to treat severe symptoms two or more times per year.

National Heart, Lung, and Blood Institute Guidelines for the Diagnosis and Management of Asthma

asthma symptoms under control, with only occasional need for quick relief. If quick-relief medications are needed on more than two days each week (not including prior to exercise), this is an indication that a change in long-term control medication may be needed.

Many of the bronchodilator and anti-inflammatory drugs used for asthma are the same ones used to treat COPD (see Chapter 4). However, they are used differently for asthma.

Other drugs sometimes used for asthma include leukotriene receptor antagonists such as montelukast (Singulair) and zafirlukast (Accolate), theophylline (Theolair, Uniphyl), cromolyn sodium (Intal), and nedocromil (Tilade).

People with severe asthma may be treated with a newer class of drugs known as biologics. These drugs target the cells causing inflammation, and include omalizumab (Xolair), mepolizumab (Nucala), and reslizumab (Cinqair). Biologics have changed the lives of many patients with severe asthma. However, they are extremely expensive, and they are not easy to dose, so patients must be closely monitored while using these drugs.

The severity of asthma can change over time, either for better or worse. Therefore, treatment may need to be adjusted either to improve control of the disease or, if it is well controlled, to attempt to reduce medications (to minimize the risk for side effects).

All medications used in asthma, and the frequency of their use, depends largely on the severity of the disease. Asthma is classified as intermittent or persistent, and persistent asthma is further classified as mild, moderate, or severe.

Intermittent Asthma

People with intermittent asthma (see Box 5-6, "Intermittent Asthma") generally only require a quick-relief medication. In most cases, this will be a bronchodilator, specifically a short-acting inhaled beta-agonist, such as albuterol (Ventolin, Proventil, ProAir, VoSpire ER), levalbuterol (Xopenex HFA), or pirbuterol (Maxair Autoinhaler). The medication is taken as needed for immediate relief when symptoms arise. People with asthma who experience symptoms during exercise may be instructed to use a short-acting inhaled beta-agonist about 10 minutes before exercising to prevent symptoms.

If a bronchodilator is needed on more than two days a week (not including exercise), it may signal that asthma is worsening or not under good control. If this happens, asthma may be classified as persistent, and a change in treatment may be warranted.

Mild Persistent Asthma

For people with persistent asthma, daily treatment with a long-term controller-type medication is used. For those with mild persistent asthma (see Box 5-7, "Mild Persistent Asthma"), this will most likely be a low dose of an inhaled corticosteroid. In addition, a short-acting beta-agonist will be used for immediate symptom relief.

Other options for long-term controller medications in people with mild persistent asthma are leukotriene receptor antagonists, theophylline, cromolyn sodium, or nedocromil.

The two leukotriene receptor antagonists (montelukast and zafirlukast) are taken in pill form, rather than inhaled. Leukotrienes are chemicals that are part of the body's natural immune system. Along with a substance called histamine, they cause inflammation in response to a perceived invader. In people with allergies and asthma, the body mistakenly perceives harmless substances, such as pollen and other allergens, as a threat. Exposure to allergens sparks leukotrienes to produce inflammation. Montelukast and zafirlukast work by blocking the action of leukotrienes, thereby preventing inflammation.

Cromolyn sodium and nedocromil, which are inhaled, are in a drug class called mast cell stabilizers. Mast cells are part of the body's immune system. In the presence of a foreign invader, mast cells break down and release large amounts of histamine, which contributes to the production of inflammation. Cromolyn sodium and nedocromil work by preventing mast cells from breaking down. This stops histamine from being released, and prevents inflammation.

Moderate Persistent Asthma

For moderate persistent asthma (see Box 5-8, "Moderate Persistent Asthma"), there are two options for long-term controller therapy:

- A medium dose of an inhaled corticosteroid, or
- A low dose of an inhaled corticosteroid, plus a long-acting inhaled beta-agonist.

If a long-acting inhaled beta-agonist is used, it should not be used as the only medication, and it should be used for the shortest possible time. Long-acting beta-agonists include salmeterol (Serevent), formoterol (Foradil), and arformoterol (Brovana). The Food and Drug Administration (FDA) issued the following statement regarding the use of long-acting beta-agonists to treat asthma. These drugs should:

- Only be used in combination with an asthma controller medication, such as an inhaled corticosteroid.
- Be used for the shortest time possible to bring asthma symptoms under control, and then discontinued.
- Only be used long-term in patients for whom asthma control cannot be achieved with other drugs.
- Be used by children and adolescents only in the form of combination drugs that contain both a long-acting beta-agonist and a corticosteroid.

In making its decision, the FDA cited studies showing an increased risk of severe worsening of asthma symptoms, leading to hospitalization and even death in some children and adults. Some studies have indicated that using an inhaled corticosteroid in combination with a long-acting beta-agonist abolishes the risk, but this has not been proven and continues to be studied. The warning does not apply to people with COPD.

The two most commonly used long-acting beta-agonists are salmeterol and formoterol. Four drugs that combine a long-acting beta-agonist with an inhaled corticosteroid are available and include salmeterol plus fluticasone (Advair), formoterol plus budesonide (Symbicort), formoterol plus mometasone (Dulera), and vilanterol plus fluticasone (Breo Ellipta).

BOX 5-8

Moderate Persistent Asthma

- Symptoms are experienced daily.
- Nighttime awakenings from symptoms occur more than once per week.
- There is a daily need for a bronchodilator (short-acting beta-agonist) for symptom relief.
- There is some limitation in normal activity.
- FEV1 is between 60 and 80 percent of predicted.
- The FEV1/FVC ratio is reduced below normal.
- Oral steroids are required to treat severe symptoms two or more times per year.

National Heart, Lung, and Blood Institute Guidelines for the Diagnosis and Management of Asthma

BOX 5-9

Severe Persistent Asthma

- Symptoms of asthma occur throughout the day.
- Awakenings from symptoms occur nightly.
- Use of a bronchodilator (short-acting beta-agonist) for symptom relief is necessary several times per day.
- There is extreme limitation in normal activity.
- FEV1 is less than 60 percent of predicted.
- The FEV1/FVC ratio is reduced below normal.
- Oral steroids are required to treat severe symptoms two or more times per year.

National Heart, Lung, and Blood Institute Guidelines for the Diagnosis and Management of Asthma

Alternatively, for moderate persistent asthma, a leukotriene modifier or theophylline may be given with a low dose of an inhaled corticosteroid. In any case, a short-acting beta-agonist will continue to be used for immediate symptom relief.

Severe Persistent Asthma

Severe persistent asthma (see Box 5-9, "Severe Persistent Asthma") is treated with a medium-to-high dose of an inhaled corticosteroid combined with a long-acting inhaled beta-agonist. Just as with moderate persistent asthma, use of a long-acting beta-agonist without an inhaled corticosteroid is not recommended.

If this does not adequately control asthma symptoms, one of three biologics—omalizumab (Xolair), mepolizumab (Nucala), or reslizumab (Cinqair)—may be used. Omalizumab binds an antibody that causes allergic reactions, thereby reducing the body's sensitivity to allergens. Omalizumab is used only in people who have moderate-to-severe asthma that is triggered by allergies. It is given by injection every two to four weeks. Mepolizumab and reslizumab reduce levels of cells called eosinophils, which play a role in allergic reactions and contribute to inflammation. These drugs are given by injection every four weeks. All the biologics are used only in combination with other asthma medications.

People with severe asthma that cannot be controlled with any of these therapies may be given oral corticosteroids. This practice is generally recommended only for short periods of time, due to the potential side effects of taking corticosteroids in pill form rather than inhaled.

Recommendations for All Asthma Patients

Once a treatment plan has been established, patients with asthma should visit their healthcare professional every one to six months (depending on the severity of their asthma) to ensure that treatment is working and that the treatment goals are being met.

This cannot necessarily be assumed. One study found that 49 percent of asthma patients were not using needed controller medication. Of the 51 percent of asthma sufferers who were using controller medications, only 14 percent had adequate control of their asthma. People with poor asthma control are at higher risk for emergency department visits and hospitalizations. Another study found that children with poorly controlled asthma had lower-quality schoolwork and more sleep problems than children with well-controlled asthma.

Improving the control of asthma symptoms has clear benefits for both children and adults. The challenge is how to accomplish this. People with moderate-to-severe asthma must set aside time from busy lives to take controller medication every day. It is easy to forget, but receiving reminders can help, and a variety of smartphone and tablet apps are available to aid with this.

It is also wise to make sure your vitamin D levels are normal, as high levels of vitamin D have associated with better lung function, and a better response to drug therapy with inhaled corticosteroids. See Chapter 7 for foods that contain vitamin D, and information on supplementing vitamin D.

Gastroesophageal reflux disease (GERD)—which causes acid to back up from the stomach into the esophagus, causing heartburn and other symptoms—can also interfere with asthma control.

Everyone with asthma should take an active role in managing and monitoring their condition by using medications as prescribed, keeping track of the frequency and intensity of symptoms, identifying triggers, and recognizing early signs that asthma may be worsening (see Box 5-10, "Your Role in Managing Your Asthma"). You may be instructed in how to use a peak flow meter to keep track of your lung function at home (see Box 5-11, "How to Use A Peak Flow Meter"). At visits to the physician's office, spirometry will often be used to test your lung function.

Immunotherapy

If your asthma symptoms are clearly triggered by identifiable allergens, immunotherapy may be recommended. Immunotherapy ("allergy shots") involves repeated injections of small amounts of the allergen (the substance triggering the reaction) in an attempt to desensitize the body to the substance. Immunotherapy is most effective in people who have a reaction to a single allergen, particularly dust mites, animal dander, or pollen.

Allergy shots can be given to children over age five and adults of all ages, even older adults. A recent study that tested allergy shots in adults ages 65 to 75 found them to be both safe and effective.

Traditional allergy immunotherapy is called subcutaneous immunotherapy (SCIT). Before immunotherapy is begun, skin tests are performed to clearly identify the allergen. First, allergy shots are given under the skin once or twice a week for about four to six months. For the next four to six months, the shots are given every two to four weeks. This therapy generally continues for several years. Eventually the body becomes less sensitive to the allergen, reducing the chance of asthma attacks.

In rare cases, a severe and potentially life-threatening reaction called anaphylaxis can occur as a result of the shots. For this reason, it is important that the shots be administered in a physician's office that is equipped with the facilities and trained personnel to treat this type of reaction.

For people with grass or ragweed allergies who don't like shots, there is another option: With sublingual immunotherapy (SLIT), small tablets are placed under the tongue, where they dissolve and are absorbed into the body. The pills are taken once a day. It must be started three to four months before exposure to the allergic substance. For a person with a pollen allergy, this means starting to use the sublingual tablets well in advance of pollen season.

Three sublingual treatments are available: Grastek (for grass pollen allergies), Oralair (for grass pollen allergies), and Ragwitek (for ragweed allergies).

Like with the allergy shots, a severe allergic reaction (anaphylaxis) can occur. Therefore, the first dose of the sublingual tablets must be taken in the doctor's office.

BOX 5-10

Your Role in Managing Your Asthma

- Identify triggers that worsen your asthma symptoms (such as allergens, irritants, tobacco smoke, etc.), and try to avoid them.
- Take all medications as directed.
- Learn the correct inhaler technique (see Chapter 4).
- Use devices, such as a spacer or nebulizer, as recommended.
- Monitor your own condition to assess how well controlled your asthma is.
- Monitor your symptoms, using a peak flow meter if prescribed.
- Recognize the signs and symptoms that suggest your asthma is worsening.
- Keep a written log to track daily actions needed to control your asthma, medications you take, and adjustments to your medication regimen.
- See your health care provider regularly, and when appropriate in response to a worsening of symptoms.

BOX 5-11

How to Use a Peak Flow Meter

A peak flow meter can be used to monitor your lung function at home. Begin by determining your baseline reading, and keep a log to compare future readings. This will help you and your doctor to know how well your treatment regimen is keeping your asthma under control. The log also can be helpful in showing cause and effect between symptoms and specific asthma triggers.

A peak flow meter is a simple hand-held device that is easy to use. For best results:

1. Stand up straight.
2. Inhale as deeply as possible.
3. Place the peak flow meter in your mouth, with your tongue under the mouthpiece and your lips closed around it.
4. Blow out as hard and fast as you can.
5. Write down the number on the peak flow meter.
6. Repeat these steps three times.

Write down the highest number in your log. To determine your baseline, take a peak flow reading every day for a few weeks while feeling your best and not experiencing any asthma symptoms. The highest number is your personal best. A subsequent reading that is 80 to 100 percent of this will be in the normal range.

The exact number of people afflicted with bronchiectasis is not known, largely because it tends to be excluded from studies that assess the incidence of obstructive airway diseases.

Bronchiectasis is a chronic obstructive airway disease in which the bronchi become damaged and easily collapse. Bronchi walls contain elastic and muscle fibers, which allow the bronchial tubes to expand and contract while maintaining their shape. In people with bronchiectasis, the elastic and muscular components in the walls of medium-sized bronchi are permanently destroyed. This damage causes the bronchi to collapse, especially with exhalation, which interferes with the ability to breathe. There are several possible causes, but bronchiectasis most often occurs following a respiratory infection.

Bronchiectasis may affect only one or two areas of the lung, or it may be more widespread. Affected areas become inflamed and possibly scarred. The smaller bronchioles beyond the affected bronchi may be destroyed. The abnormally dilated bronchi then have severely impaired ability to clear mucus, and the excess mucus that builds up in the lungs can harbor bacteria or other infectious agents. This may lead to a vicious cycle of a respiratory infection that damages the bronchi, which causes dilation of the bronchi, and impairs their ability to clear mucus. The excess mucus traps bacteria, thus continuing the infection and causing additional damage to the bronchi.

Very rarely, infants and children can develop bronchiectasis from a birth defect that impedes the normal development of the lungs. The disease more often affects adults or children who have suffered a chronic or recurring lung infection, or who have an inherited lung disease called cystic fibrosis.

The exact number of people with bronchiectasis is not known, largely because it tends to be excluded from studies that assess the incidence of obstructive airway diseases. It is known to be more common in women than in men, and its prevalence increases with age. For unknown reasons, Native Americans living in Alaska are four times more likely than the general population to have bronchiectasis.

What Causes Bronchiectasis?

Bronchiectasis may occur in people who've had poorly treated or untreated lung infections, such as tuberculosis, pertussis, or severe bacterial pneumonia. Measles, whooping cough, influenza, fungal infections, mycobacterial infections, and adenovirus infection are other possible causes. Bronchiectasis due to scarring as a result of severe infection is uncommon in the United States and other developed countries, partly because of the widespread use of antibiotics and other effective treatments for these infections. Bronchiectasis due to slowly progressive lung infections—especially from organisms often referred to as atypical mycobacteria—does occur in the developed world.

Bacteria
The most common bacterial family to cause bronchiectasis in this manner is mycobacteria. Worldwide, *Mycobacterium tuberculosis*,

the bacteria that causes TB (see Chapter 9), is a common cause of bronchiectasis. In the U.S., other non-communicable mycobacteria (atypical mycobacteria) are more common causes of bronchiectasis. Of these, the bacteria *Mycobacterium avium* is the most commonly found. Interestingly, these bacteria tend to affect smokers with emphysema and older, thin, non-smoking Caucasian women more than other groups. Scientists have no idea why these patients seem more susceptible to these bacteria.

Obstructions

Obstruction of bronchial tubes can also be a cause of bronchiectasis. For example, an inhaled object (such as unchewed food or a small toy) can lodge in the airways, causing an obstruction. This obstruction may lead to an infection, with subsequent development of bronchiectasis. Enlarged lymph nodes, a tumor in the lung, or a mucus plug (see Box 6-1, "Bronchiectasis") can also cause an obstruction that leads to bronchiectasis.

Cystic Fibrosis

Cystic fibrosis is an inherited disease in which an abnormal gene causes mucus to be too thick and sticky. Mucus builds up in the lungs, creating an obstruction. These obstructions are called mucus plugs. Most people with cystic fibrosis develop severe bronchiectasis as a result of the airway obstruction from mucus plugs and chronic lung infection.

Other Causes

Other possible causes of bronchiectasis include a genetic condition called Young syndrome that is similar to cystic fibrosis, and a rare inherited disorder called primary ciliary dyskinesia, which causes poor mucus clearance and recurring lung infections. People with a compromised immune system, particularly when it results from deficiency in a protein called immunoglobulin, are also susceptible to bronchiectasis. People with alpha-1 antitrypsin deficiency may develop bronchiectasis, as can those with autoimmune diseases such as rheumatoid arthritis, Sjögren's syndrome, or inflammatory bowel disease, particularly ulcerative colitis. Exposure to toxic gas, such as chlorine gas or ammonia, also may cause bronchiectasis.

Symptoms of Bronchiectasis

Symptoms of bronchiectasis usually begin slowly, following a respiratory tract infection. A longstanding (months

BOX 6-1

Bronchiectasis

Normal Airway

Airway with Bronchietasis

to years) daily cough with sputum production is the chief symptom. Some people will cough up small amounts of blood as a result of damage to the airways from infection. People with bronchiectasis may also have shortness of breath, wheezing, chest pain, fever, weakness, and weight loss. Sometimes, the condition produces relatively few symptoms.

Many people with bronchiectasis suffer repeated bouts of lung infections (bronchitis, pneumonia) that require antibiotics.

Diagnosing Bronchiectasis

Because the symptoms of bronchiectasis can be similar to those of other lung diseases such as asthma, COPD, and pneumonia, a physician will look for the conditions associated with bronchiectasis, such as recurring or untreated lung infections or cystic fibrosis. If bronchiectasis is suspected, the sputum that is produced from coughing will be examined for the presence of white blood cells (a sign of infection), and may be sent for culture to see if a predominant bacterium is present.

A computed tomography (CT) scan may be used to confirm the diagnosis and to determine the extent of the disease. Pulmonary function tests such as spirometry are not necessary to make the diagnosis, but may be performed to assess the severity of the disease by measuring lung function. Additional tests may be performed to identify the underlying cause. This is important because some causes of bronchiectasis require specific treatments.

Treatment for Bronchiectasis

The treatment for bronchiectasis partly depends on the underlying cause of the condition. General recommendations for all patients with bronchiectasis include limiting exposure to inhaled toxins, such as air pollution and secondhand smoke. Those who smoke should quit. Immunizations for influenza and pneumonia are recommended. Getting adequate nutrition is essential, and may require taking nutritional supplements. Medications may be used.

Overall, the treatment for bronchiectasis is effective, and people with the disease have the same life expectancy as people with asthma or COPD. Those with cystic fibrosis are the exception, due to the severity of the bronchiectasis that occurs, and due to its unique cause.

Medications

Antibiotics are an important treatment for most people with bronchiectasis. Antibiotics that may be used include amoxicillin (Amoxil), tetracycline (Sumycin), trimethoprim-sulfamethoxazole (Bactrim, Septra), and azithromycin (Zithromax), among others. Antibiotics are usually given for seven to 14 days, but may be given for longer periods to prevent infections from coming back.

In some circumstances, antibiotics also may be prescribed to be inhaled through a nebulizer. Generally, this is done to decrease the amount of bacteria that grows in the airways of patients with bronchiectasis. Some doctors prescribe the inhaled antibiotic to be taken every day. Other physicians prescribe the antibiotic to be taken daily every other month.

Bronchodilators and corticosteroids may be used in some patients with bronchiectasis, but there is no conclusive evidence that these are beneficial for everyone with the condition.

Mechanical Methods

Mechanical methods may be used to help clear large amounts of mucus that can build up in the lungs. A person with bronchiectasis may undergo postural drainage with percussion or vibration. Postural drainage entails being placed in position with the head and/or chest down to allow the force of gravity to help clear the mucus. This may be combined with percussion, in which a healthcare professional will tap the chest with a cupped hand for about one to two minutes. This can help to break up thick mucus.

A procedure called vibration may also accompany postural drainage. This involves a healthcare professional placing his or her hand on the patient's chest and creating vibrations. Vibration is also often done using a special vibrating vest. Other devices that may be used to help clear mucus include flutter devices, intrapulmonic percussive ventilation devices, acapella devices, and incentive spirometry.

Surgery

Surgery to remove damaged parts of the lung may be an option for some bronchiectasis patients. Surgery is generally reserved for patients in whom the lung damage is confined to, or markedly more severe in, a specific area rather than spread throughout the lungs, and who are not helped with antibiotics.

Some people with severe bronchiectasis, such as advanced cystic fibrosis, may be candidates for lung transplantation.

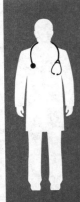

Most people recover from the flu without incident. But young children and older adults are at risk for developing complications from the flu.

Influenza—commonly called "the flu"—is a viral infection of the respiratory system. It affects the lungs, as well as the whole body. Most people recognize the symptoms—fever, body aches, sore throat, stuffy nose, and headache. Sometimes the flu is confused with the common cold, but while some flu symptoms are the same as those of a cold, these are different illnesses caused by different viruses. In general, the flu is more severe. It's often possible to continue going about your daily activities with a cold, but the flu usually causes a fever and extreme exhaustion that necessitate bed rest for a few days. Some people with gastrointestinal symptoms like nausea and vomiting call their illness "stomach flu." However, the flu rarely causes these symptoms. "Stomach flu" symptoms are more likely to occur in children than adults.

You get the flu by breathing in the influenza virus through the nose or mouth. When someone who has the flu coughs, sneezes, or even talks, droplets containing the virus are expelled into the air, and can be breathed in by people nearby. The flu virus can also be picked up by touching an object that has been contaminated by someone with the flu. Touching an infected surface and then moving your hand near your face allows the virus to be inhaled through the nose or mouth (see Box 7-1, "Practical Tips to Avoid Catching or Spreading the Flu").

Most people who get the flu come down with it during "flu season," which runs from November to March. Children are more susceptible to getting the flu, and often spread the virus to others. Most people recover from the flu, with or without treatment, within a week or so, but the flu is unpredictable, and its severity varies from year to year.

Three Types of Flu

There are three types of influenza virus: A, B, and C. Types A and B are more common, and usually lead to more severe symptoms than type C. Type C influenza is most likely to affect children younger than age six. Most people develop immunity to influenza C early in life, and if they subsequently come in contact with the virus, it causes only mild or no symptoms. The viruses that cause more suffering and lead to flu outbreaks are types A and B. The genes of these viruses change over time, and different strains circulate each year.

Flu Symptoms

Infection with the influenza virus causes the lining of the respiratory tract to become swollen and inflamed. The infection is in the respiratory system, but symptoms are felt throughout the body. Symptoms generally appear one to four days after becoming infected. They start abruptly and usually include fever (100°F to 102°F), body aches, weakness, and extreme exhaustion. Some people may experience headache or cough, and others may have a sore throat, stuffy nose, and sneezing. The fever usually subsides in two to three days, but full recovery takes about a week. Children with the flu have the same symptoms as adults, but they tend to have higher temperatures (103°F to 105°F).

BOX 7-1

Practical Tips to Avoid Catching or Spreading the Flu

Vaccines for prevention are advised. However, the Centers for Disease Control and Prevention also offer practical advice to avoid getting or spreading the flu:

- Cover your nose and mouth with a tissue when you cough or sneeze. Throw the tissue in the trash after you use it.

- Wash your hands often with soap and water, especially after you cough or sneeze. If soap and water are not available, use an alcohol-based hand rub that is at least 62 percent alcohol.

- Thoroughly wash towels, eating utensils, and dishes of the person with the flu before they are shared with anyone else.

- If you get the flu, stay home from work or school and limit contact with others to keep from infecting them.

- Avoid touching your eyes, nose, or mouth.

The flu is diagnosed on the basis of symptoms and whether other cases of flu have been reported in the community. Laboratory tests are generally not necessary, but may be done in some cases to determine the type of influenza virus responsible for an epidemic.

Complications from Flu

Most people recover from the flu without incident. However, complications can arise in children younger than age five, older adults, pregnant women, and people with a chronic disease (including asthma and COPD) or a weak immune system. These people are most likely to be hospitalized or die from the flu.

Having the flu can temporarily alter the immune system, making the lungs susceptible to a bacterial infection that can lead to pneumonia. The flu virus itself also can cause pneumonia. Typically, pneumonia symptoms appear after flu symptoms start to go away. The sudden appearance of a high fever, chest pain, and coughing that produces thick, yellow-greenish-colored mucus are signs of pneumonia. Other infections that may occur as a result of the flu include sinusitis, bronchitis, and ear infection.

People with heart disease and/or a lung disease such as COPD or asthma can experience a worsening of their condition when they get the flu. Annual flu vaccines are recommended for everyone at risk for complications from the flu.

Some people who get the flu become seriously ill, and may even die. For example, during the 2009-2010 flu season, the strain of the influenza virus responsible for most cases of the flu was called pandemic H1N1 (also called "swine flu." Pandemic means that it occurred over a wide geographic area, and affected a large number of people). Most people infected with this virus had only mild symptoms, but others became seriously ill and died. Many of those who died were healthy young adults, who generally have the lowest risk for serious illness and death from the flu.

The H1N1 strain reappeared in 2013-2014, but did not cause a pandemic, largely because many people had been exposed to it during the first outbreak and developed immunity against it. Different strains dominated the 2014-2015 flu season. In particular, the H3N2 virus was particularly hard on older adults, resulting in the highest rate of flu-associated hospitalizations among people age 65 and older since 2005. The 2015-2016 flu season was relatively mild.

Treatment for Flu

Antiviral medicines are available to treat the flu, but they must be taken within the first 48 hours of becoming sick in order to be effective. They should be taken for at least five days. The antiviral drugs—oseltamivir (Tamiflu) and zanamivir (Relenza)—don't completely cure the flu, but they may reduce the length of the illness and lessen the symptoms. One study found that zanamivir can shorten the duration of symptoms by about one day, and reduce infections that sometimes develop after the flu. The two medications work against both influenza types A and B.

Zanamivir generally is not recommended for people with COPD or asthma, because studies have found that some people with these conditions develop bronchospasm (wheezing) after taking this drug. If zanamivir is used by someone with COPD or asthma, a fast-acting inhaled bronchodilator should be available to immediately relieve bronchospasm.

Some flu symptoms can be treated with over-the-counter medications, but these products do not treat the viral infection and will not shorten the length of illness. Aspirin can be used to bring down a fever, but it should not be used in children younger than age 18, since children and teenagers who take aspirin when they have the flu are at risk for developing Reye's syndrome, a condition that affects the nerves. While this is an uncommon complication, it is not worth the risk. Use of acetaminophen (Tylenol) in children does not appear to be linked to Reye's syndrome, and is therefore preferred for reducing a fever.

Decongestants and antihistamines can be used for relief of cough, stuffy nose, and other nasal symptoms. It's also advisable to drink plenty of fluids and to rest.

Vaccination for Flu

The best defense against the flu is yearly vaccination. The ideal time to get a flu shot is in October or November, just as the flu season is getting started. But it's never too late: Vaccination is recommended any time during the season. A recent study found that getting the flu shot in the morning may provide more protection for older adults than if it's given later in the day. However, if the afternoon or evening is the only time you have to get vaccinated, do so—it will still be effective.

The flu vaccine consists of killed particles of the influenza virus. These particles do not cause the illness, but instead prime the body to recognize the virus and to make antibodies against it. Antibodies are molecules made by white blood cells that bind to an infectious agent and render it harmless. If a vaccinated person is exposed to the influenza virus, the antibodies usually destroy the virus before symptoms appear. After vaccination, it takes about two weeks for the antibodies that protect against infection to develop in the body.

A higher dose version of the flu vaccine, called Fluzone High-Dose, is available for people age 65 and older. It contains four times the amount of antigen (the killed virus particles that stimulate the immune system) than the regular vaccine. This creates a stronger protective response that should be beneficial for older adults, who have weaker immune systems than younger people.

Vaccination works only if the body creates antibodies against the correct strain of the virus. Because influenza viruses constantly change over time, vaccine makers must develop new flu vaccines each summer by predicting the strain of flu expected to be most prevalent in the coming season. Nearly two years in advance of a flu season, they must make an educated guess about which types will appear in order to produce enough flu vaccine for everyone. Because it is impossible to guess 100 percent correctly, the vaccine does not protect against every strain of the virus that appears. However, it does protect against enough strains to save thousands of lives and prevent countless individuals from getting sick.

Who Should Get a Flu Shot?

Everyone can benefit from getting a flu shot, and the Centers for Disease Control and Prevention (CDC) recommend vaccination for everyone six months of age and older.

Most people have little or no reaction to the flu shot. A few people may develop swelling or soreness at the injection site, and a smaller number of people may experience a day or two of headache and mild fever. For people age 65 and older, Medicare covers annual flu shots, including the high-dose version. Many health insurance plans also pay for flu shots.

People who don't like getting shots have a second option for vaccination: an influenza vaccine called FluMist, which is administered as a nasal spray. This vaccine is made with a live but weakened virus, but has been approved by the Food and Drug Administration only for healthy people between the ages of two and 49. Last year, the CDC recommended against Flu-Mist for both adults and children (see Box 7-2, "CDC Says 'No' to Flu-Mist").

The benefits of vaccination have been demonstrated over and over. One study found that getting the seasonal flu vaccine cut flu-related hospitalizations among older adults by nearly two-thirds. Even if the flu shot doesn't completely prevent the flu in everyone, it most likely prevents the most serious side effects of the flu. Getting vaccinated against the flu can also lessen the severity of pneumonia, if it occurs

A study found that babies born to women who get a flu shot during pregnancy are less likely to be underweight when born, and have fewer respiratory illnesses during flu season.

Who Should Not Get a Flu Shot?

Influenza vaccinations are helpful for most people, but some people should avoid getting them. These include:

- Infants younger than six months
- Anyone with an acute illness and fever. Wait until you're feeling better before getting vaccinated.

Special Considerations for Flu Shots

In the past, people with an allergy to eggs were advised against getting a flu shot, because the flu vaccine is grown in chicken eggs. In 2017, the CDC advised that people with egg allergy be given age-appropriate inactivated flu vaccine or recombinant flu vaccine. If they have had an allergic reaction to eggs more severe than hives, they should get the shot at their doctor's office or other location where they can be supervised by a healthcare provider. They can also opt for Flublok, which does not use chicken eggs in its manufacturing process. It is approved for use in adults age 18 and older.

People who ever had Guillain-Barre syndrome (a rare disorder of the nervous system) should talk to their doctor about the flu shot. Some people who have this condition should not get a flu shot.

Vitamin D

Some research suggests that getting adequate amounts of vitamin D may strengthen the immune system and lessen your chances of getting the flu. Vitamin D is found in salmon, mackerel, tuna, and fortified milk and juice. Many people meet their vitamin D requirement through exposure to the sun. Others require vitamin D supplements. The recommended daily intake is now 1,000 international units (IUs) of vitamin D3 (cholecalciferol), which is stronger and more active than vitamin D2 (ergocalciferol).

NEW FINDING   BOX 7-2

CDC Says "No" to Flu-Mist

When given a choice between a shot and a nasal spray, most people would pick the nasal spray. But in the case of Flu-Mist, an influenza vaccine may from weakened live flu virus, the CDC recommends against using this product in children and adults. Although use of a live virus sounds dangerous, the opposite is true: Compared with flu shots, the Flu-Mist was much less effective during the 2013-2014 and 2015-2016 flu seasons, primarily because it offered insufficient protection against the H1N1 influenza virus.

Annals of Internal Medicine, February 7, 2017

LUNG INFECTIONS

The air we breathe contains numerous germs. Once these are inhaled, the body has several mechanisms for expelling and destroying them—for example, hair-like projections (cilia) in the bronchial tubes work together with mucus to rid the lungs of foreign invaders that may cause harm. In addition to this mechanical defense, the body's immune system has the ability to destroy germs. Sometimes, however, the body's natural defenses are unable to fight off viruses, bacteria, fungi, or other germs, and they cause a respiratory infection such as influenza, pneumonia, or tuberculosis.

Pneumonia is an infection in one or both lungs caused by bacteria, virus, or other infectious agent. The severity of pneumonia depends on several factors, including which germ is responsible and the strength of the individual's immune system.

When the immune system detects an infection, it produces inflammation, which triggers processes designed to promote healing. For example, inflammation creates a barrier around the infected area to prevent the germ from spreading. In addition, chemical factors are produced that attract immune system cells to the area to fight the infection. Inflammation in the lungs can also cause coughing, difficulty breathing, and other pneumonia symptoms.

When alveoli (tiny air sacs in the lungs) become inflamed they fill with pus and other fluids. The body tries to clear this through coughing. The alveoli are the location in the lungs where oxygen passes into the bloodstream, so when the alveoli are inflamed, oxygen can't easily enter the bloodstream (see Box 8-1, "Pneumonia"). Too little oxygen combined with spreading infection, which can occur in people with a weakened immune system, can lead to death. About 55,000 Americans die of pneumonia each year.

Pneumonia is usually treated and cured with antibiotics in young and healthy adults, but it is more common and can be harder to cure in people age 65 and older. One study found that older adults hospitalized for pneumonia are at increased risk for cognitive impairment, depression, and physical disability, meaning that effective prevention and treatment are especially important. Pneumonia is also harder to cure in infants and young children, people with chronic health problems (such as heart disease, lung disease, or diabetes), and anyone with a weakened immune system. Several diseases can weaken the immune system, including HIV/AIDS. People taking chemotherapy for cancer, or taking drugs to suppress the immune system after an organ or bone marrow transplant, also have weakened immune systems.

Some people get pneumonia after a bout of the flu or a cold. People at high risk for this include the following:

- Young children
- Pregnant women
- Older adults
- People with chronic health conditions, such as asthma, diabetes, heart disease, or lung disease.

The lungs have five lobes, three in the right lung and two in the left. The infection can affect a part of a lobe, an entire lobe, or several lobes. Pneumonia that affects one or more lobes is called lobar pneumonia. Pneumonia can also affect patches throughout a lung, in which case it is called bronchial pneumonia.

When pneumonia is contracted outside of a hospital or other healthcare setting, it is called community-acquired pneumonia. In the United States, about four million people get this type of pneumonia each year, mostly in the winter.

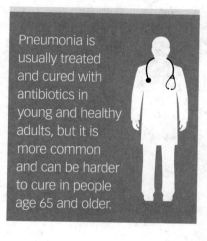

Pneumonia is usually treated and cured with antibiotics in young and healthy adults, but it is more common and can be harder to cure in people age 65 and older.

BOX 8-1

Pneumonia

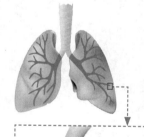

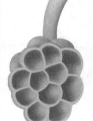

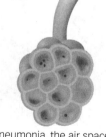

Healthy alveoli

In pneumonia, the air space is filled with fluid and pus containing bacteria and blood cells, and the alveoli walls are swollen. This limits the exchange of oxygen with carbon dioxide, making breathing difficult.

© Alila07 | Dreamstime.com

Pneumonia that occurs during a hospital stay for some other illness is called hospital-acquired pneumonia. People on a mechanical ventilator (a machine that helps you breathe) are especially at risk for this type of pneumonia. This can occur when bacteria passes down the breathing tube into the lungs.

What Causes Pneumonia?

Infectious agents that can cause pneumonia include bacteria, viruses, fungi, and mycoplasmas (a type of bacteria that lack a cell wall). These germs are all around us, in the air we breathe and, in the case of some types of fungi, in the soil. They generally don't make us sick, because the body's natural defenses eliminate or destroy them. However, if the immune system is weakened for some reason, the germs can enter the lungs, where they multiply and cause pneumonia.

Bacterial Pneumonia

The most common cause of pneumonia is infection with one of dozens of different types of bacteria. The most common bacterium responsible for bacterial pneumonia is *Streptococcus pneumoniae* (also called *pneumococcus*). Older adults, people with chronic illnesses, and other people in the high-risk categories listed above may develop bacterial pneumonia after having the flu or a cold.

Bacterial pneumonia can be serious and even life threatening, especially if bacteria pass into the bloodstream and spread to other parts of the body.

Viral Pneumonia

Viruses also can cause pneumonia. Children younger than age five are particularly susceptible to viral pneumonia. Adults with heart or lung disease, and women who are pregnant are more likely than other adults to develop this type of pneumonia. In adults, influenza is the most likely cause of viral pneumonia. Other viral culprits are respiratory syncytial virus, rhinovirus, and herpes simplex virus, among others. Patients taking medications that suppress the immune system are at high risk of developing viral pneumonias, especially from a virus called cytomegalovirus.

Viral pneumonia is often milder than bacterial pneumonia, and some people get better in a few weeks, even without treatment. However, it can also be serious, require treatment, and sometimes be fatal, especially in those who have a weakened immune system due to medications or other serious medical conditions, like cancer or liver disease.

Mycoplasma Pneumonia

Mycoplasmas are bacteria that lack a cell wall. Mycoplasma pneumonia occurs most commonly in people younger than age 40. People with this type of pneumonia generally have only mild symptoms, and they respond well to treatment with antibiotics. It is rarely fatal.

Fungal Pneumonia

Certain types of fungi can cause pneumonia in susceptible people. These fungi include three found in soil: *coccidioidomycosis* in southern California and the desert Southwest, *histoplasmosis* in the Ohio and

Mississippi River Valleys, and *cryptococcus*. *Pneumocystis jiroveci* (formerly called *Pneumocystis carinii*) is a yeast-like fungus that can also cause pneumonia. This is often referred to as *pneumocystis pneumonia*.

When healthy people are exposed to these fungi, they generally do not develop pneumonia or other serious illness. People with weakened immune systems, especially people with HIV/AIDS or cancer, or those taking medications that suppress the immune system, are most at risk for developing pneumonia from these organisms.

Aspiration Pneumonia

Another type of pneumonia occurs when a substance in the mouth (such as food, drink, vomit, or saliva) is inhaled into the lungs (aspirated). Occasionally, people with gastroesophageal reflux disease (GERD) may develop aspiration pneumonia when small amounts of gastric contents are refluxed into the back of the throat or the mouth, and subsequently inhaled.

Symptoms of Pneumonia

Symptoms of pneumonia vary depending on a number of factors, such as the organism causing the pneumonia, the type of pneumonia (lobar or bronchial), the person's overall health, and whether pneumonia follows the flu or a cold.

Symptoms of pneumonia that is caused by bacterial infection tend to appear suddenly, and usually include fever and difficulty breathing (see Box 8-2, "Pneumonia Symptoms").

In people who develop pneumonia as a consequence of the flu, symptoms like cough, fever, and sore throat generally appear suddenly, after flu symptoms have gone away.

The symptoms of viral pneumonia usually start more gradually than those of bacterial pneumonia, and often mimic flu symptoms (fever, cough, headache, muscle aches, and weakness). Difficulty breathing increases as the disease progresses. Symptoms of viral pneumonia often are milder than those of bacterial pneumonia, but they can still be severe.

Diagnosing Pneumonia

In people with the symptoms described above, the doctor will take a medical history and perform a physical examination. The doctor will then use a stethoscope to listen to the chest for characteristic crackling, bubbling, and rumbling sounds (called "rales") that may indicate the presence of infection in the lungs.

If pneumonia is suspected, a chest X-ray will be performed. The X-ray can reveal the presence of pneumonia and its location in the lungs. It cannot be used to determine the organism causing the infection.

A blood sample will most likely be taken for a type of blood test called a complete blood count (CBC). This shows the number of white blood cells in the blood sample. White blood cells are part of the body's immune system response. A high number of white blood cells in the sample may indicate the presence of a bacterial infection. A blood culture may also be performed. This test determines the presence of bacteria in the bloodstream, and is used to find out if the infection has spread outside the lungs.

BOX 8-2

Pneumonia Symptoms

Common Symptoms
- Chest pain when breathing or coughing
- Fever
- Shaking chills
- Cough
- Shortness of breath
- Wheezing
- Green mucus (in severe cases)

Less Common Symptoms
- Nausea
- Vomiting
- Diarrhea
- Loss of appetite

For Pneumonia Prevention, See Your Dentist

It may sound strange, but people who never see a dentist have twice the risk of bacterial pneumonia than those who get dental checkups twice a year, a study has found.

The link between dental care and pneumonia in critically ill patients is well known. This study of more than 26,650 patients across the U.S. looked at the connection in the general population, and found it to be equally strong.

The connection does not surprise infectious disease specialists, who say that the direct conduit between the mouth and the lungs makes it easy to aspirate bacteria. Those most likely to be affected were white, older (average age 47), likely to have comorbidities and cognitive limitations, and less likely to have dental insurance.

Presented at Infectious Disease Week, October 2016

To identify the exact organism causing the infection, a sputum test may be performed. In this test, phlegm that is coughed up is analyzed under a microscope to identify the microorganism infecting the lungs.

Treatment for Pneumonia

Treatment for pneumonia depends on the cause and severity of the illness. In many cases, a person with pneumonia can rest at home while undergoing treatment. More severe cases may require a stay in the hospital. Pneumonia caused by bacteria or mycoplasmas will be treated with antibiotics. Antibiotics may be given as pills that can be taken at home. In more serious cases, antibiotics may be administered intravenously during a stay in the hospital, or started in the hospital for a few days and continued at home. Severe cases of pneumonia may also necessitate treatment with oxygen, which will most likely be administered in the hospital.

Commonly prescribed antibiotics are not effective against viral pneumonia. Certain kinds of viral pneumonia can be treated with specific antiviral medications, but in many cases, viral pneumonia is treated with rest and plenty of fluids. Antifungal medications are used to treat pneumonia caused by fungal infection.

After a few days of taking antibiotics or antiviral medications, a person with pneumonia should start to feel better. The length of time for full recovery will depend on the severity of the pneumonia, and the overall health of the individual. In otherwise healthy people, the acute infectious phase of pneumonia is cured in one to two weeks. However, complete healing of the damaged lung may take an additional two to four weeks. It is extremely important to continue taking any prescribed medications for the entire length of time prescribed, even if symptoms subside. Failing to do so may allow the microorganism to reestablish itself, and lead to a recurrence of pneumonia.

Everyone with pneumonia should get plenty of rest, eat a healthy diet, and drink lots of fluids, since fluids help to loosen the mucus in their lungs.

Preventing Pneumonia

Because pneumonia tends to occur in people with a weakened immune system, staying as healthy as possible is the best way to prevent it. Eat a nutritious diet, exercise regularly, avoid smoking, and try to reduce stress.

Recently, regular dental care was found to cut the risk of bacterial pneumonia (see Box 8-3, "For Pneumonia Prevention, See Your Dentist").

Vaccines are available against the most common cause of pneumonia (*Streptococcus pneumoniae*). A vaccine called Prevnar 13 protects against 13 subtypes of these bacteria. A different vaccine, called Pneumovax 23, protects against 23 subtypes. All adults age 65 and older should receive both of these vaccines, but they can't be given at the same time. Prevnar 13 is usually given first, and Pneumovax 23 is given one year later. Prevnar 13 is also recommended for infants and children ages two months to five years. Pneumovax 23 is recommended for adults ages 19 to 64 who smoke or have asthma. Unlike the flu shot, which must be given every year, pneumococcal vaccination provides protection for at least five years and can be given at any time of the year.

People at high risk of developing pneumonia as a complication of influenza should get a yearly flu shot.

TUBERCULOSIS

Tuberculosis (TB) is a contagious disease that usually attacks the lungs. Before effective treatment became available in the 1940s, TB (which was formerly known as consumption) killed many people. In fact, in the early 1900s one out of every seven people in the United States died of TB. The disease also killed many prominent people, including Emily Bronte, Anton Chekov, George Orwell, and D.H. Lawrence.

In the late 1800s and early 1900s, people with TB were often sent to sanatoriums, where they were exposed to cold air and sunshine, which were thought to be therapeutic. In the 1940s, the treatment of TB was revolutionized by the discovery of antibiotics effective against TB. The disease slowly declined but did not completely go away, and the number of cases in the U.S. began to rise in 1985.

Measures to reverse this trend resulted in the lowest number of cases (9,412) ever reported in 2014. The number of cases remains level, but has not dropped further.

The rate of TB remains 13 times higher among people born outside the U.S. In the U.S., the rate of TB is 29 times higher among Asians, and eight times higher among blacks and Hispanics, than among whites.

Some people with TB have developed a strain of the disease that is resistant to the antibiotics used to treat it. Additionally, success in treating and preventing TB in the U.S. has not been mirrored around the world, and the disease continues to be a major cause of death in several countries.

TB is caused by infection with a bacterium called *Mycobacterium tuberculosis*, which is contracted when bacteria expelled from the lungs by coughing, sneezing, or exhaling are inhaled. TB usually affects the lungs, but it may also affect other organs.

TB is not easily transmitted because a person with TB only expels a small amount of bacteria into the air. Repeated exposure to someone with TB for weeks or months is usually necessary for transmission to occur. That's why only about one-third of people who are exposed to TB become infected. TB is most commonly passed among people who live or work close together.

It's important to understand the difference between infection with TB (sometimes called "latent" TB) and active TB disease (see Box 9-1, "Symptoms of Tuberculosis"). People who breathe in the bacteria can become infected, but only about 10 percent of people who become infected develop active disease. Only people with active disease can transmit the disease to others.

TB Infection

When TB bacteria are breathed in, they pass through the airways to the alveoli. The immune system goes to work to protect the body from these bacteria. White blood cells called macrophages engulf and kill many of the bacteria, but the cell walls of TB bacteria

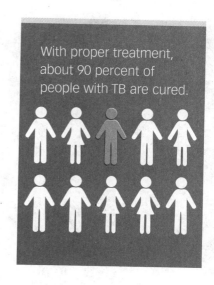

With proper treatment, about 90 percent of people with TB are cured.

BOX 9-1

Symptoms of Tuberculosis

Latent TB does not cause any symptoms. A person with active TB may have some or all of the following symptoms:

- Persistent cough
- Fatigue
- Weight loss
- Fever
- Night sweats
- Loss of appetite
- Coughing up blood

If TB spreads to other parts of the body, symptoms depend on the organ affected. Early symptoms of active TB—like fatigue, fever, and weight loss—may be vague, and may mimic other diseases. Therefore, anyone who has been exposed to someone with TB should get tested.

are resilient, and they protect some bacteria from being killed. The immune system identifies macrophages containing these live bacteria, and creates a wall around them. The resulting lung nodules are called tubercles (see Box 9-2, "Progression of Tuberculosis"). As long as the TB bacteria remain inside the tubercles, they do not cause symptoms, and do not spread. These bacteria can remain inactive for months, years, or even decades. This dormant infection is called non-contagious latent TB. About 90 percent of people with latent disease never have active disease, and the bacteria eventually die.

Active Tuberculosis Disease

Some people with TB infection develop active disease. If the immune system is weak, it may not have the ability to fight off the infection. Or, the TB bacteria may escape from the tubercles and spread. Left unchecked, the bacteria multiply and damage the lungs or other parts of the body. Because TB bacteria infect the alveoli (the tiny air sacs where oxygen passes into the bloodstream), bacteria can move into the bloodstream and infect the lymph nodes, bones, kidney, brain, spine, or skin. People with active disease are contagious. In people who develop active TB, the disease usually develops within a short time after infection. Some people with latent TB may develop active disease months or years later if their immune system is weakened by HIV/AIDS, diabetes, older age, alcohol or drug abuse, or chemotherapy.

Diagnosing Tuberculosis

A skin test can tell whether a person has been infected with TB bacteria. Even people with latent TB will have a positive test result. The test (called the Mantoux test) involves injecting a substance called tuberculin just under skin of the forearm. If a red bump forms at this site two to three days later, the size of the bump will determine if it indicates TB infection. If TB infection is diagnosed, this doesn't necessarily mean the person has active TB.

BOX 9-2

Progression of Tuberculosis

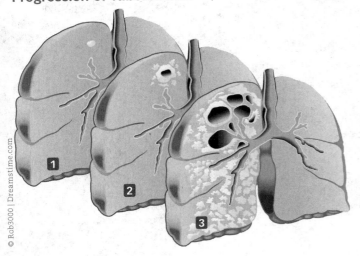

© Rob3000 | Dreamstime.com

1 Tuberculosis infection in the right upper lobe.

2 The initial plaque progresses, digging a hole.

3 Formation of numerous cavities and bronchial erosions.

To determine whether a person with TB infection has active disease, the doctor will ask about exposure to persons with TB, other health conditions, and the presence of any of characteristic TB symptoms. A chest X-ray will be performed to look for evidence of the disease in the lungs. The doctor will also take a sample of sputum (coughed-up mucus) to be tested for the presence of TB bacteria. The results of this test are also used to decide which antibiotics to use to treat the disease.

Treatment for Tuberculosis

With proper treatment, about 90 percent of people with active TB are cured. Left untreated, active TB destroys the lungs and causes death in about 60 percent of infected people. Treatment is advised even for people with latent TB, to prevent active disease, and usually involves taking the drug isoniazid once a day for nine to 12 months.

Once the disease becomes active, the treatment regimen is more complex. Drug treatment may begin during a short stay in the hospital. Medications will then be continued at home, and must be taken for six months to one year. A combination of isoniazid plus two or three other antibiotics, such as rifampin, pyrazinamide, or ethambutol will be prescribed. A few weeks after beginning these drugs, the person with active TB will start to feel better and will no longer be contagious. Even though symptoms may subside, however, it will be necessary to take the medications for the entire length of time prescribed to completely kill the bacteria. If the medications are stopped too early, the bacteria can become active again.

Additionally, if antibiotic medications are not taken consistently, the bacteria may evolve in ways that allow them to resist attack by one or more of the antibiotics. When this happens, a person is said to have drug-resistant TB. If bacteria are resistant to one antibiotic, the person often can be given other drugs that kill TB bacteria. However, some people have what's called multidrug-resistant TB (MDR-TB), because the TB bacteria they are infected with have developed resistance to two or more drugs. Extensively drug-resistant TB (XDR-TB) is virtually untreatable with any of TB drugs.

MDR-TB is very difficult to cure. It requires taking special drugs capable of killing bacteria that have developed resistance against most antibiotics. These drugs tend to have serious side effects, and treatment may be required for up to two years. Even with treatment, it is estimated that about half of people with MDR-TB will die. MDR-TB can also be passed from person to person, making prevention especially important. The most effective way to prevent MDR-TB is to take all medications as directed for the entire length of time they are prescribed.

Addiction: A physiologic need for a habit-forming substance, such as alcohol, nicotine, or certain drugs.

Airways: The tube-like organs of the respiratory system through which air is breathed in and out. These include the trachea, bronchi, and bronchioles.

Allergen: A substance that is not a harmful infectious agent, yet can trigger a response by the immune system. Some common allergens are animal dander, plant pollen, and mold. An allergic reaction can lead to an asthma attack.

Alveoli: These are tiny air sacs clustered at the end of the smallest bronchial tubes (bronchioles) in the lungs. The primary function of the lungs—the exchange of carbon dioxide and oxygen—takes place in the alveoli. The walls of the alveoli are extremely thin and surrounded by capillaries (tiny blood vessels). This allows for carbon dioxide to pass easily from the blood in the capillary into the alveoli, and for oxygen to travel from the alveoli through the capillary wall and into the bloodstream.

Aorta: The large, main artery exiting the heart. All blood pumped out of the left ventricle travels through the aorta on its way to other parts of the body.

Artery: Blood vessels that carry oxygenated blood from the heart to the organs and tissues.

Bacteria: Single-cell organisms that exist everywhere on earth, including inside plants and animals. There are numerous types of bacteria; many have beneficial functions, but some cause infectious diseases. These include Streptococcus pneumoniae, and Mycobacterium tuberculosis.

Beta-adrenergic receptor: Muscle cells that surround the bronchial tubes contain a particular type of receptor called beta-adrenergic receptors. A receptor is a group of molecules embedded in the wall of a cell. When another molecule attaches to this receptor it causes the cell to undergo a change. When stimulated (by a neurotransmitter or pharmaceutical drug) these receptors cause the muscle cell to relax, which opens constricted airways.

Bronchial tubes: Inside the lungs, a branching system of bronchial tubes carry air from the trachea into the tiny air sacs (alveoli) where oxygen and carbon dioxide are exchanged. The larger bronchial tubes are called bronchi and the smaller ones bronchioles (See Alveoli).

Capillaries: The smallest of the body's blood vessels, these deliver nutrients and oxygen to the body's cells and remove wastes like carbon dioxide from the cells.

Carbon dioxide (CO_2): A colorless, odorless gas that is a waste product of bodily processes of humans and other animals. It is removed from the body via the lungs, through exhalation. Carbon dioxide in the air is absorbed by plants and used during photosynthesis.

Cholinergic receptor: A cholinergic receptor causes muscle cells to constrict. In the lungs this means that airways will become constricted and narrowed. Blocking the action of this receptor has the opposite effect; it opens up the airway (See Beta-adrenergic receptor).

Cilia: These are tiny hair-shaped cells that project from the lining of several organs in the body. For example, they are present in the trachea, where they beat in coordinated waves to sweep particles out of the body, thus preventing them from entering the lungs.

Circulatory system: Composed of the heart, blood, and blood vessels (veins and arteries), the circulatory system distributes blood throughout the body. Blood that contains oxygen (oxygenated) is pumped from the lungs into the heart and out through the arteries to all parts of the body. Veins carry blood that has been depleted of oxygen back to the heart where it is pumped into the lungs to receive oxygen.

Diaphragm: A sheet of muscle shaped like a dome that extends across the bottom of the rib cage, just below the lungs. As this muscle contracts and relaxes, it assists with the act of breathing by helping to draw air into the lungs and push air back out again.

Exacerbation: A worsening or increased severity of a disease.

Exhalation: The movement of air (containing carbon dioxide) from the lungs out into the environment through the mouth and nose.

Fungus (plural: fungi): These organisms include mushrooms, molds, yeast, and mildews. They range in size from a single cell to a larger mass. They often have spores that grow a network of slender tubes called hyphae. Some fungi, such as Coccidioides immitis, Histoplasma capsulatum, and Pneumocystis jirovecii, can cause infections, including pneumonia.

Gene: These are basic biological units that act as the codes which direct the creation and functioning of life. A gene is made up of DNA. DNA is composed of four types of chemicals called bases—adenine (A), thymine (T), cytosine (C), and guanine (G). A string of these bases makes up a gene. The varying combination of bases is responsible for different characteristics and physical functions, such as eye and hair color. Each person has thousands of genes, which are arranged along 23 pairs of longer structures called chromosomes. Each chromosome in a pair is inherited either from the mother or father.

Hypercapnia: The condition in which there is too much carbon dioxide (see Carbon dioxide) in the blood. It is generally caused by impaired gas exchange, often as a result of emphysema.

Hyperinflation: Excessive inflation of the lungs. People with emphysema who have hyperinflation of the lungs can develop a barrel-shaped chest.

Hypoxemia: A condition in which there is too little oxygen in the blood. The main cause is impaired gas exchange, often as a result of emphysema. If the body's tissues don't get adequate amounts of oxygen, the consequences can be severe and even life threatening.

Immune system: The immune system is a complex system that defends the body against attacks by foreign invaders. It can recognize potentially dangerous substances (such as bacteria and viruses) and mount attacks via specialized cells. In some people this system may go awry, causing harmless substances (like plant pollen or house dust) to be seen as dangerous. This may trigger an allergic reaction and possibly contribute to asthma.

Influenza: Commonly known as the flu, this is caused by coming in contact with a virus in a family of viruses called Orthomyxoviridae (influenza viruses). There are several influenza subtypes. The virus can be transmitted from person to person through coughing or sneezing or by coming in contact with body fluids (saliva, blood, nasal secretions) or contaminated surfaces. Symptoms of the flu include fever, chills, sore throat, muscle pain, weakness, and fatigue. A vaccination is available to protect against the flu.

Inhalation: The intake of air (containing oxygen) from the outside environment through the mouth and nose into the lungs.

Mucus: A thick, slippery substance that coats the inside walls of the airways (trachea, bronchi, and bronchioles). When small particles (such as dust, pollutants, allergens, or pathogens) are breathed in, they get caught in the mucus and are swept away from the lungs by tiny, hair-like cells (cilia). Mucus also helps to moisturize inhaled air, keeping the airways from drying out. The presence of mucus is normal. However, lung diseases such COPD, asthma, and bronchiectasis can cause too much mucus to be produced, which can lead to difficulty breathing.

Mucous membrane (mucosa): The layer of cells lining the inside walls of the respiratory system. Mucous membranes secrete mucus that can help prevent infection and illness.

Mycoplasma: Single-celled bacteria that lack a cell wall. One type, Mycoplasma pneumonia, can infect the upper respiratory tract and lungs, and is a major cause of lung infection and walking pneumonia in children and young adults.

Neurotransmitter: A chemical substance produced by the body that acts as a messenger in the brain and nervous system by transmitting nerve impulses from one cell to another cell, muscle, tissue, or organ; examples include dopamine, epinephrine, and serotonin. Neurotransmitters play an essential role in the normal functioning of the brain.

Nicotine: An addictive substance found in the tobacco plant that acts as a stimulant.

Oxygen: A colorless, odorless gas that makes up more than 20 percent of the volume of air. Oxygen is essential to support the life of humans, animals, and plants.

Pathogen: An organism that causes disease; common pathogens include bacteria, viruses, and fungi.

Pneumonia: Inflammation of the lungs, which is often caused by a bacterial infection; the bacteria that most commonly causes it is Streptococcus pneumoniae. Symptoms of pneumonia include cough, chest pain, fever, and difficulty breathing. Two vaccines that protect against Streptococcus pneumoniae are available and are recommended for people age 65 and older.

Pulmonary: This term refers to the lungs.

Respiratory system: Respiration is another word for breathing. The respiratory system is composed of organs that supply oxygen-rich blood to all parts of the body and also remove carbon dioxide through the act of breathing. The respiratory system includes the trachea, lungs, bronchi, bronchioles, and alveoli.

Secondhand smoke: Tobacco smoke from cigarettes, cigars, or pipes that is inhaled involuntarily from the environment by someone who is not smoking. Breathing in second-hand smoke can put people, especially children, at risk for lung disease.

Side effects: Most drugs have biologic effects in addition to the intended therapeutic effect. For example, corticosteroid drugs are very effective at reducing inflammation, but they also may cause side effects, such as cataracts, osteoporosis, muscle weakness, hair loss, mood changes, and weight gain. For most drugs, the side effects are milder than this and they may not occur in all people who take the drug. Drug manufacturers are required to list all known side effects on the medication leaflet.

Sputum: The material that is coughed up from the respiratory tract is called sputum. It is generally a mixture of mucus and saliva. A sputum sample may be obtained to detect infections in the respiratory tract.

Tolerance: In medical terminology, the word tolerance has a specific meaning. When a drug, such as nicotine or a painkiller, is taken over a long period of time, the body develops tolerance. This means that increasingly larger doses are required to achieve the same effect.

Trachea: Also called the windpipe, the trachea is a tube-like organ that begins just below the larynx (also known as the voice box) and leads into the bronchial tubes of the lungs.

Vaccination: Vaccines are weakened or killed forms of a pathogen. When a vaccine is administered the exposure causes the body to build up defenses against that pathogen. If the pathogen is encountered in the future, the immune system is ready to fight it off before it can take hold and cause disease. Vaccines are available to prevent many diseases, including common childhood diseases, such as measles and chickenpox. Vaccines are also available against influenza and pneumonia.

Veins: These are blood vessels that carry deoxygenated blood back toward the heart and lungs.

Virus: These tiny microorganisms cannot exist apart from a living cell. They infect living cells and use the internal workings of those cells to stay alive and reproduce. Viruses are responsible for many infections in humans, including the common cold (caused by the rhinovirus), the flu (influenza), AIDS (human immunodeficiency virus [HIV]), and pneumonia.

For general information about COPD, contact the following organizations:

Allergy & Asthma Network
www.allergyasthmanetwork.org
800-878-4403
8229 Boone Boulevard, Suite 260
Vienna, VA 22182

American Academy of Allergy, Asthma and Immunology
www.aaaai.org
414-272-6071
555 East Wells Street, Suite 1100
Milwaukee, WI 53202-3823

American Association of Cardiovascular and Pulmonary Rehabilitation (AACVPR)
www.aacvpr.org
312-321-5146
330 N. Wabash Avenue, Suite 2000
Chicago, IL 60611

American Association for Respiratory Care
www.aarc.org
972-243-2272
9425 N. MacArthur Boulevard, Suite 100
Irving, TX 75063-4706

American College of Allergy, Asthma, and Immunology
www.acaai.org
847-427-1200
85 West Algonquin Road, Suite 550
Arlington Heights, IL 60005

American College of Chest Physicians
www.chestnet.org
224-521-9800/800-343-2227
2595 Patriot Boulevard
Glenview, IL 60026

American Lung Association
www.lungusa.org
1-800-586-4872
55 W. Wacker Drive, Suite 1150
Chicago, IL 60601

Association of Asthma Educators
www.asthmaeducators.org
888-988-7747
70 Buckwalter Road, Suite 900, #330
Royersford, PA 19468

Asthma and Allergy Foundation of America
www.aafa.org
1-800-727-8462
8201 Corporate Drive, Suite 1000
Landover, MD 20785

Centers for Disease Control and Prevention
www.cdc.gov
800-232-4636
1600 Clifton Road
Atlanta, GA 30329-4027

National Heart, Lung, and Blood Institute Information Center
www.nhlbi.nih.gov
301-592-8573
P.O. Box 30105
Bethesda, MD 20824-0105

North American Quitline Consortium
www.naquitline.org
800-398-5489
3219 E. Camelback Road, #416
Phoenix, AZ 85018

Pulmonary Education and Research Foundation (PERF)
www.perf2ndwind.org
310-539-8390
P.O. Box 1133
Lomita, CA 90717-5133

QuitNet
www.quitnet.com

U.S. Environmental Protection Agency
Local air quality forecast
www.airnow.gov